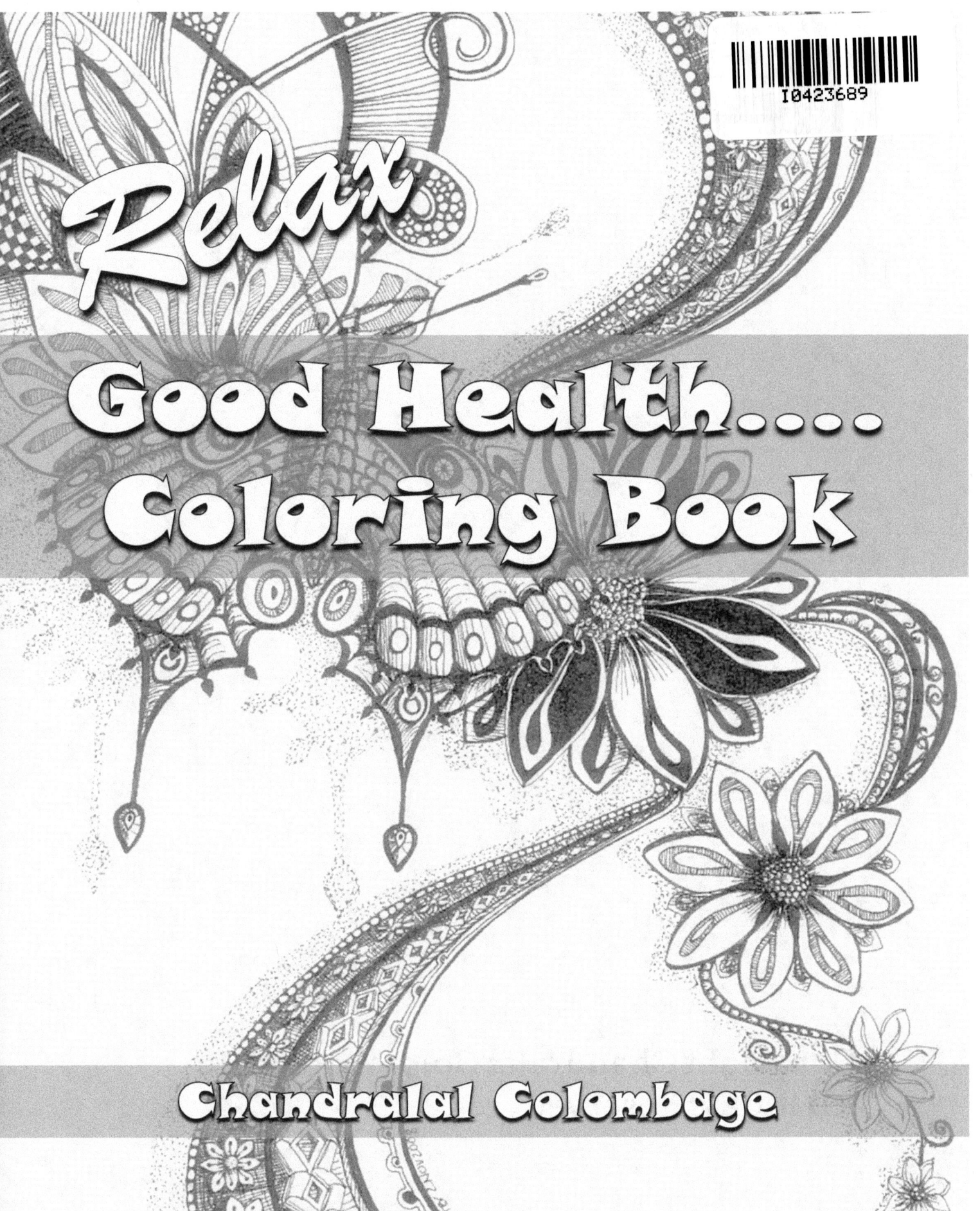

Relax

Good Health.....
Coloring Book

Chandralal Colombage

Dedication

To Good Health in all Beings and Good Fun to keep you young

I want to thank you and congratulate you for purchasing your copy of "Good Health Coloring Book".

You've probably heard of using mandalas for meditation. But have you ever heard of coloring mandalas as a therapeutic practice?

By coloring mandalas, we allow ourselves to play. By playing, we open up a broad range of creative and intuitive processes that we don't normally experience in our day-to-day lives. It is play that will always open up our spirit, and facilitate a connection to our higher understanding and purpose.

By coloring or painting these powerful symbols, we also become a part of the circle, which involves us in the cyclical nature of our bodies, our lives, our thoughts, our emotions, just about everything.

Use this page to test your colours, so you know which pencil/crayon/fibre tip pen to use, to get the colour you want.

Our greatest happiness does not depend on the condition of life in which chance has placed us, but is always the result of a good conscience, good health, occupation and freedom in all just pursuits.

Thomas Jefferson

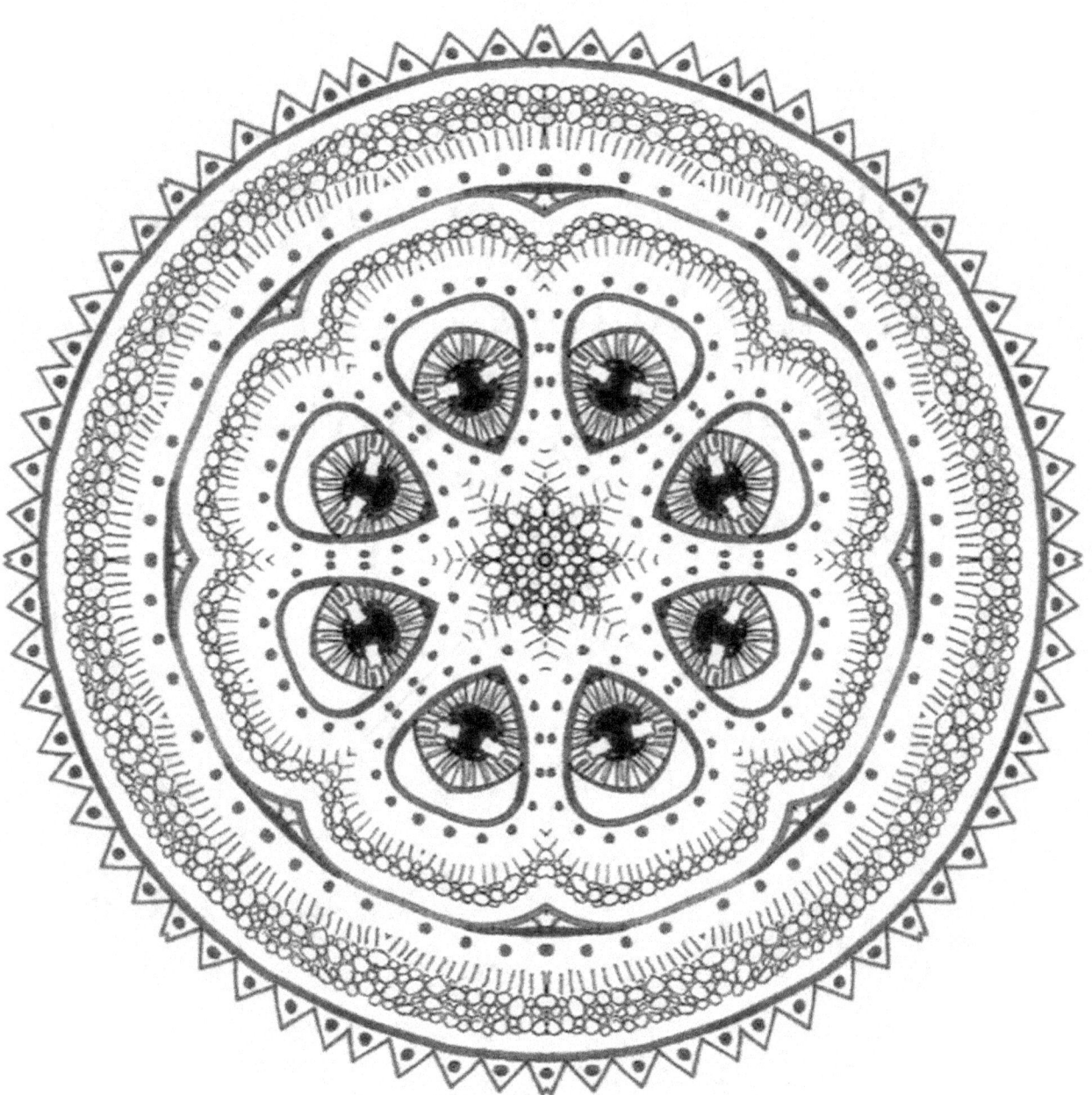

Calm mind brings inner strength and self confidence, so that's very important for good health..

Dalai Lama

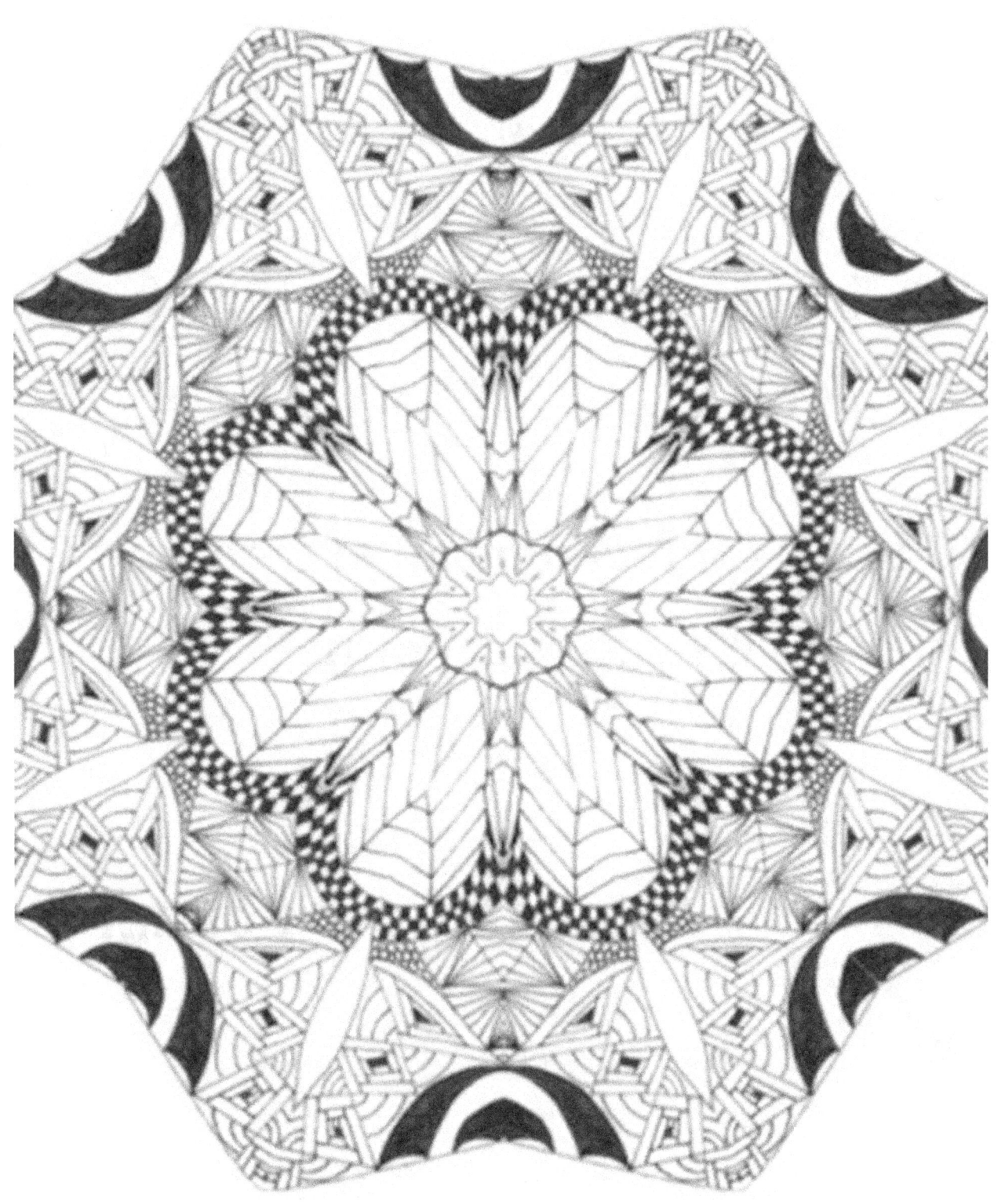

Good health is not something we can buy.

However, it can be an extremely valuable savings account.

Anne Wilson Schaef

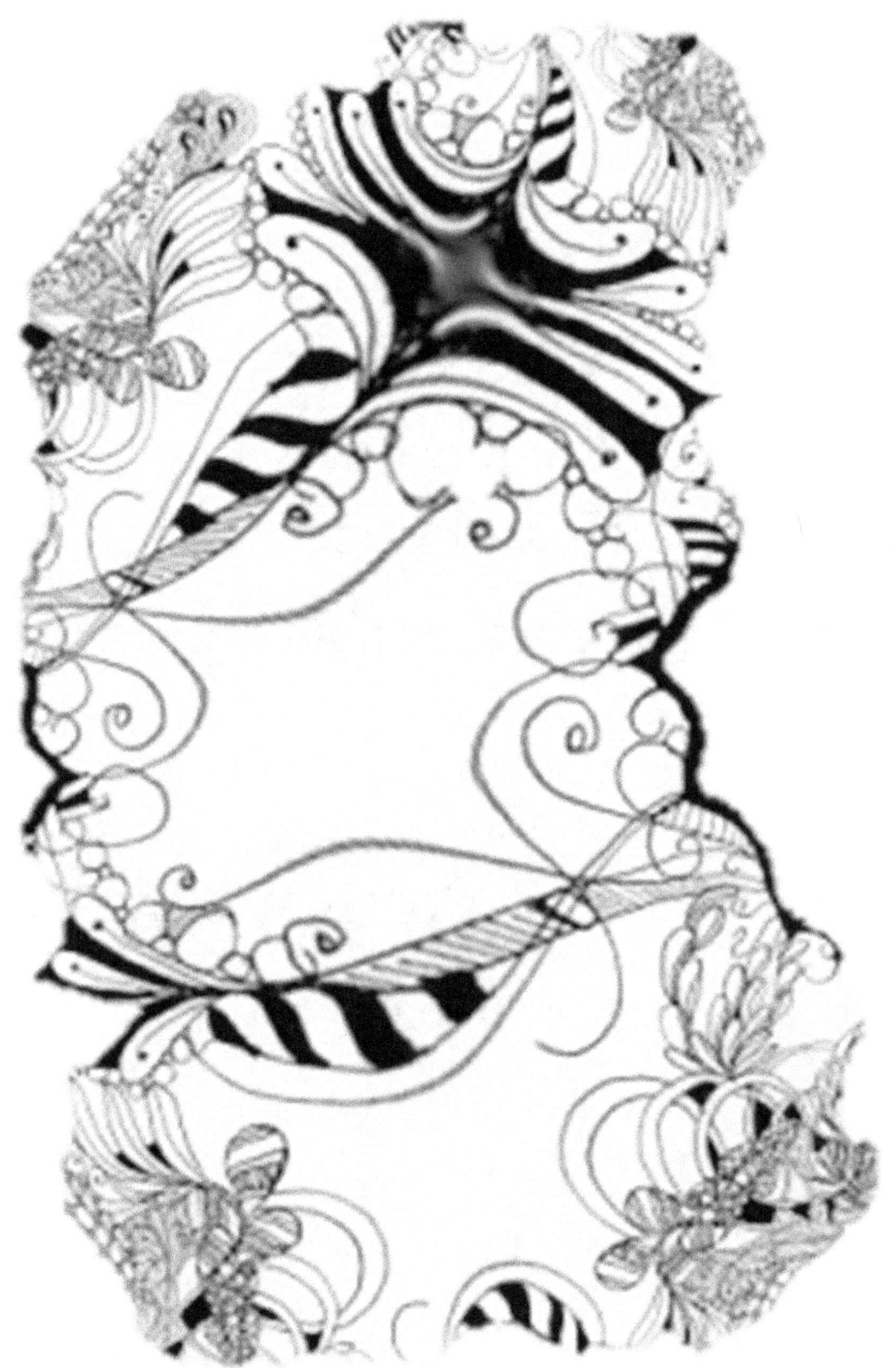

Good health and good sense are two of life's greatest blessings.

Publilius Syrus

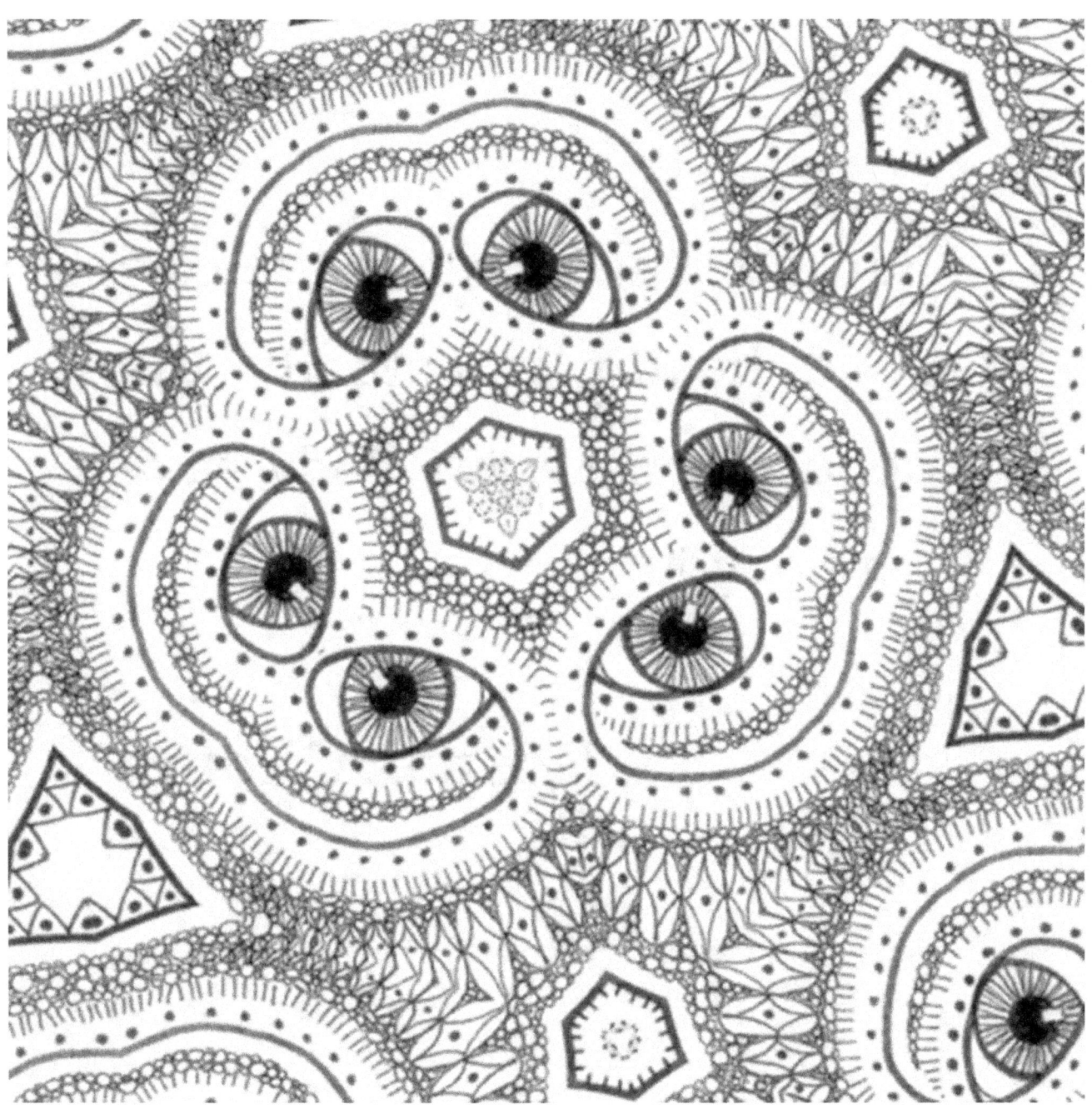

But the real secret to lifelong good health is actually the opposite: Let your body take care of you.

Deepak Chopra

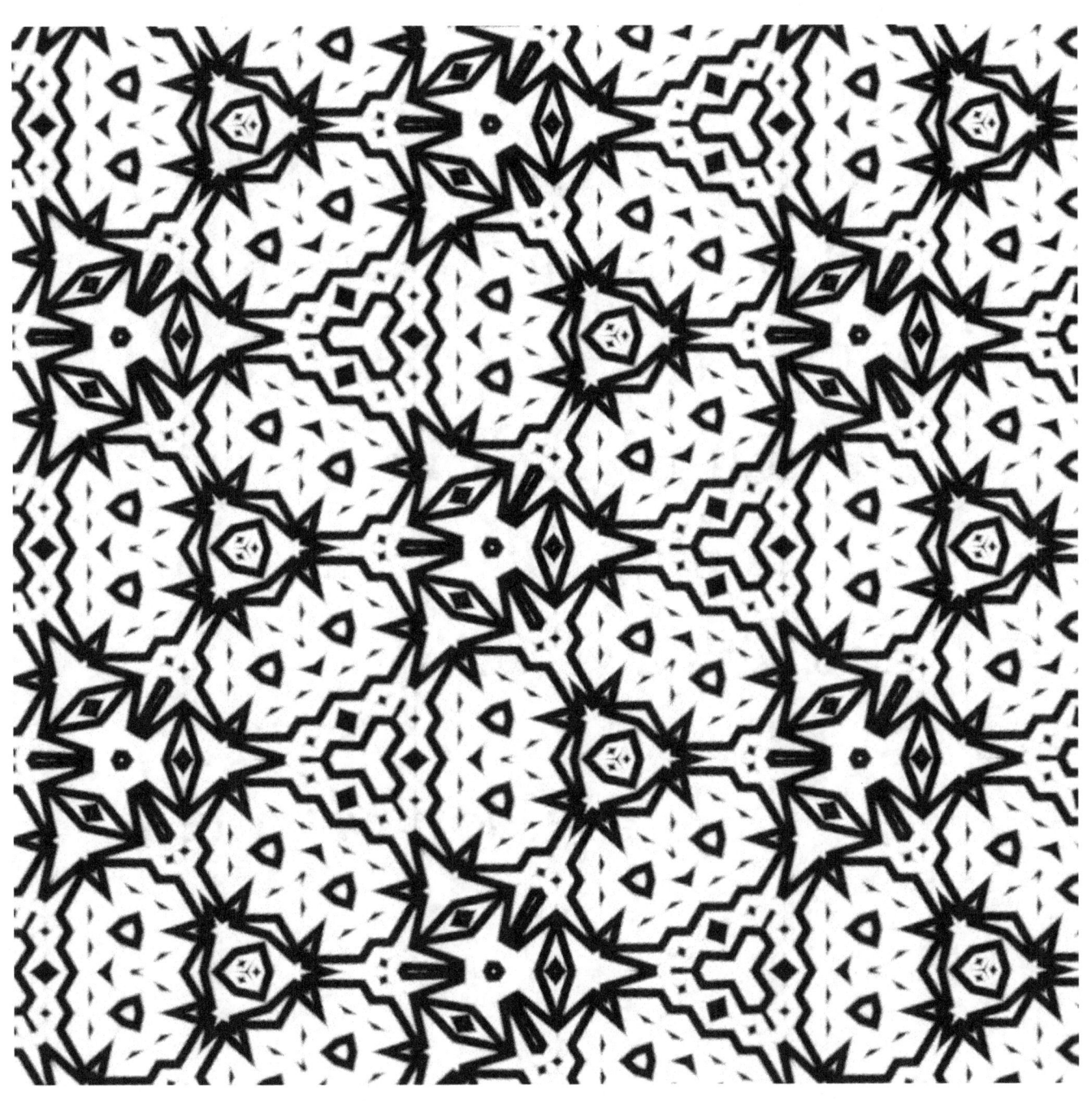

I am confident that nobody will accuse me of selfishness if I ask to spend time, while I am still in good health, with my family, my friends and also with myself.

Nelson Mandela

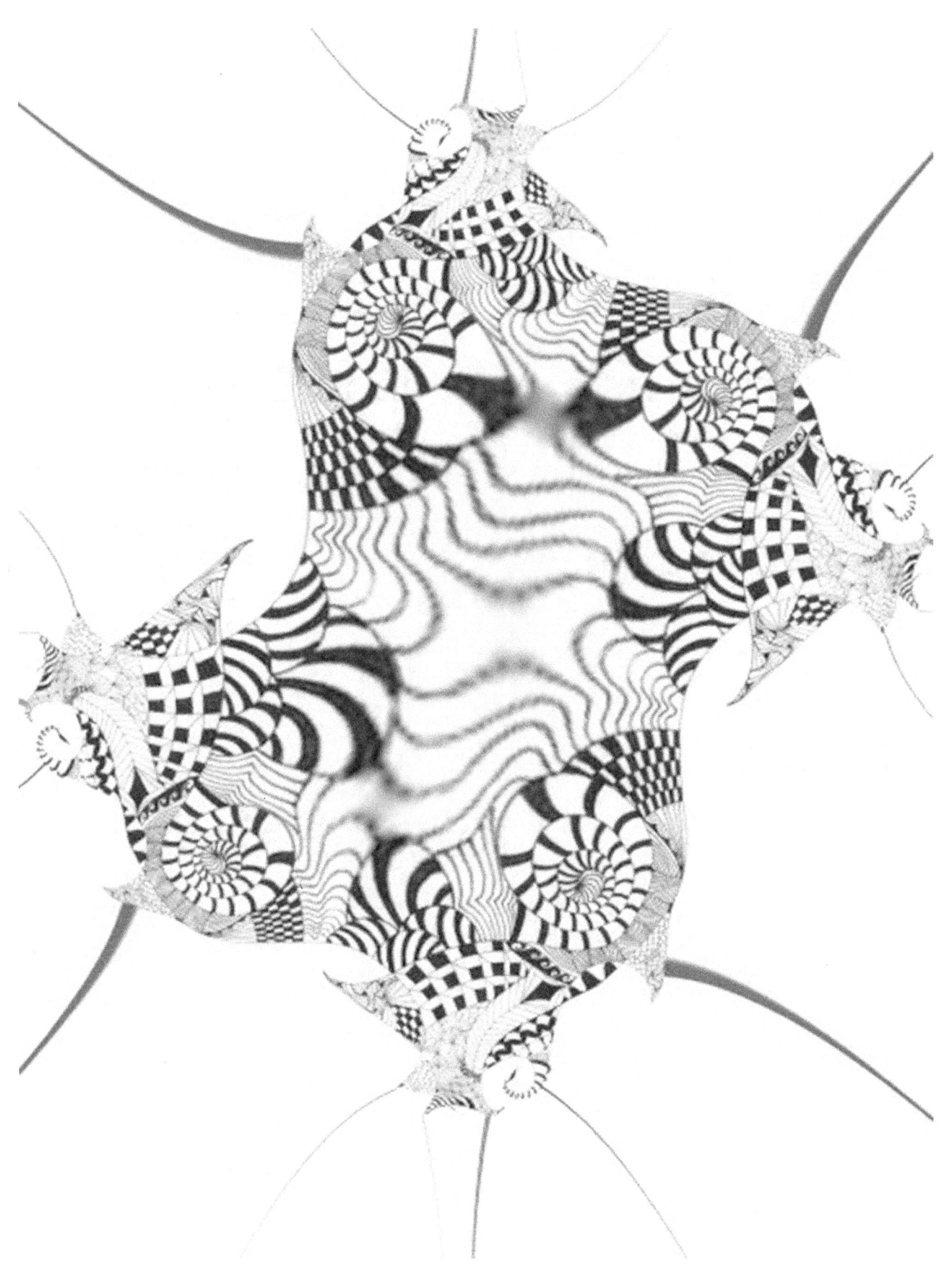

In the midst of these hard times it is our good health and good sleep that are enjoyable.

Knute Nelson

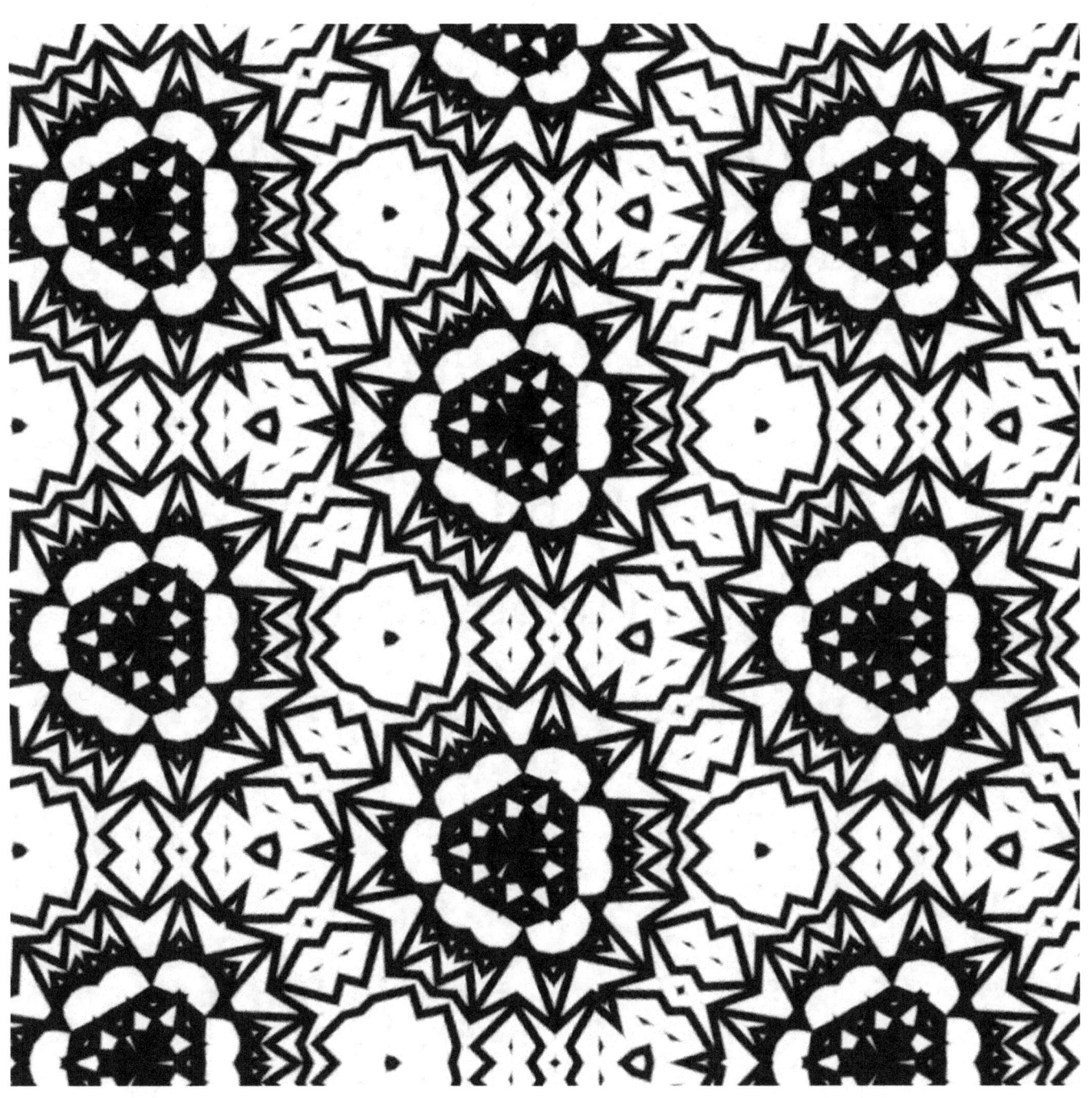

I'd be happy to live till 80 as long as I was comfortable and in good health. Mind you, ask me again on the eve of my 80th birthday.

Even so, I hope we don't all start living to be 120. I'm not sure I'd cope with another 60 years.

Bonnie Tyler

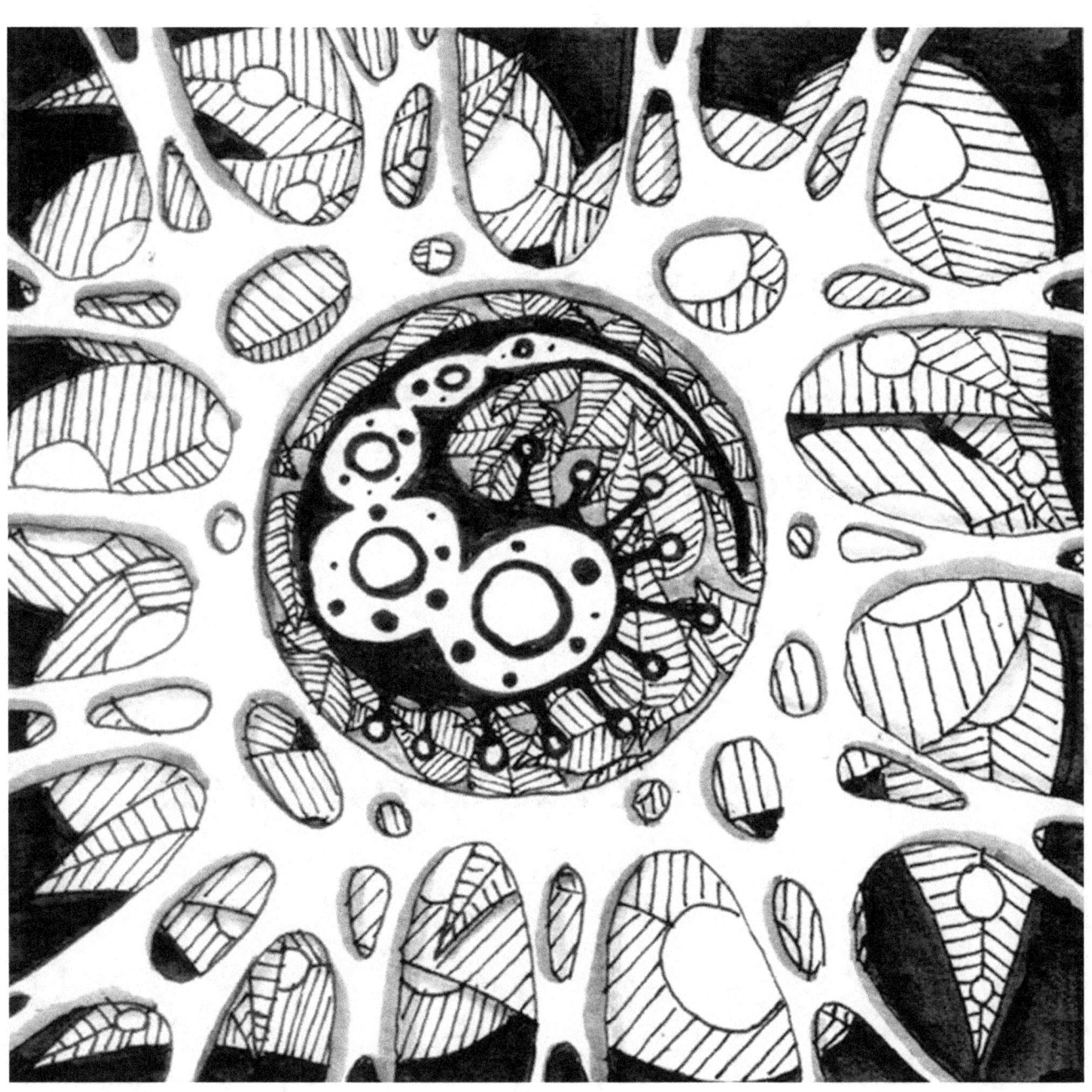

Happiness is nothing more than good health and a bad memory.

Albert Schweitzer

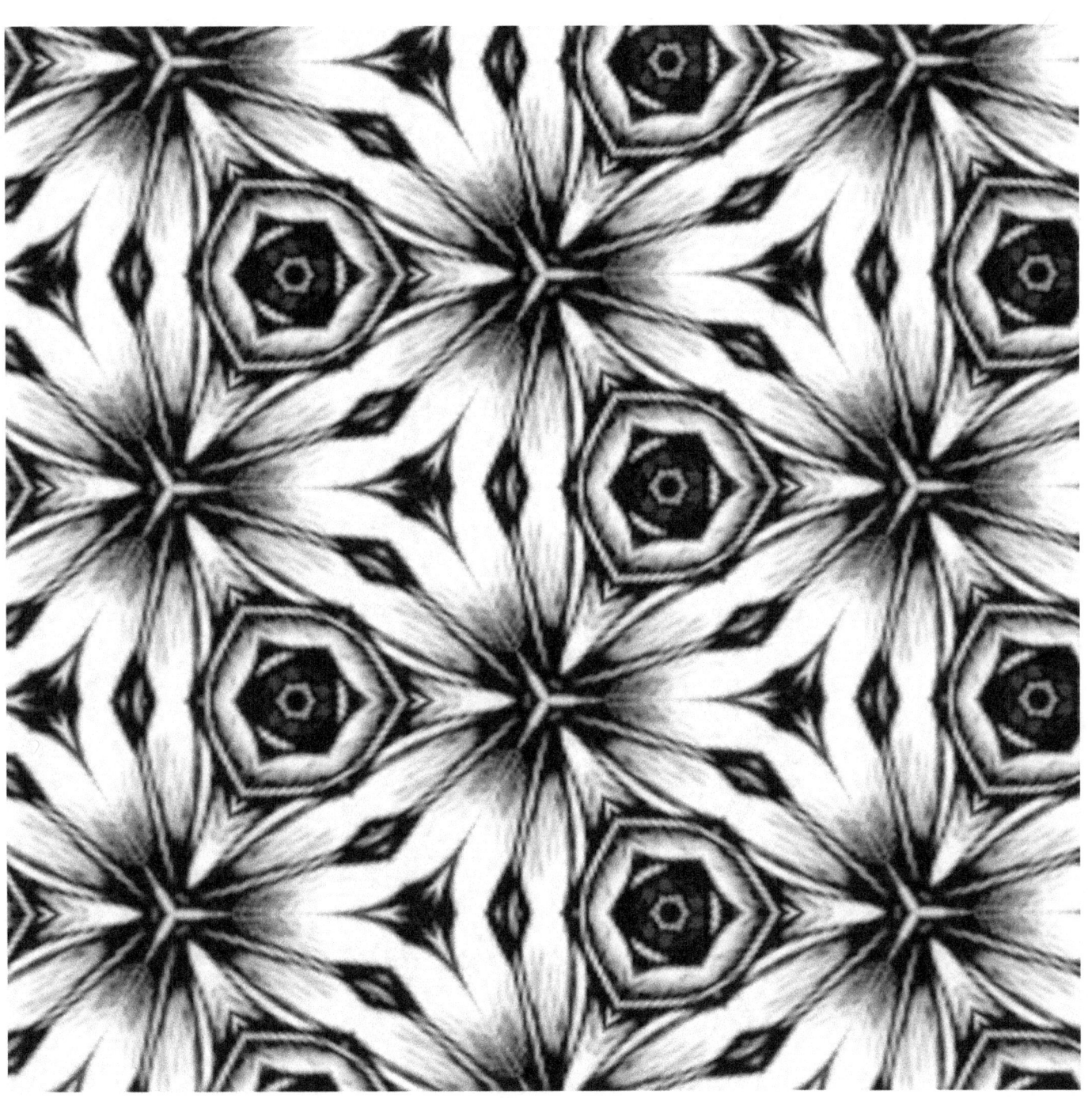

To enjoy the glow of good health, you must exercise.

Gene Tunney

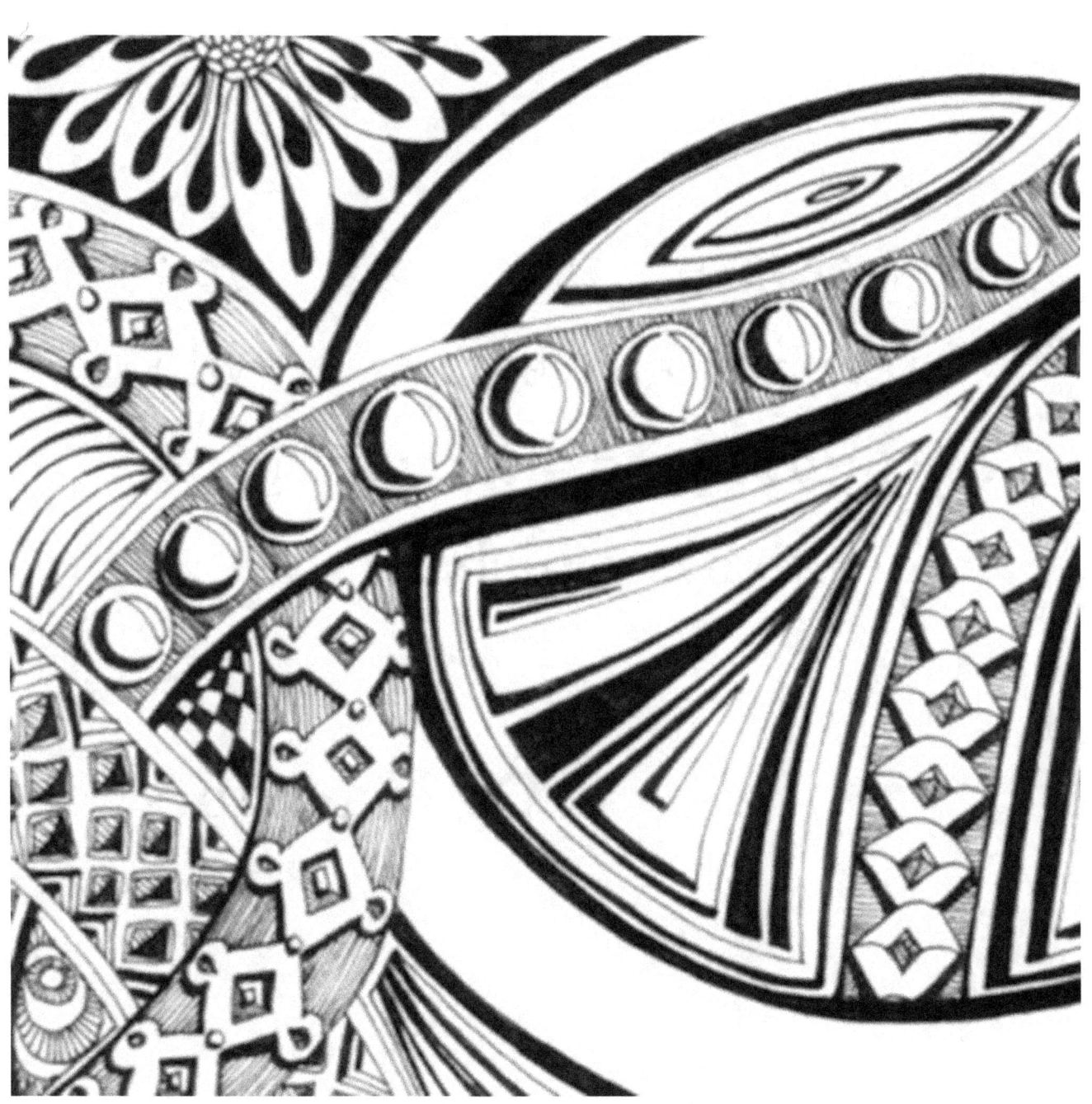

Treasure the love you receive above all. It will survive long after your good health has vanished.

Og Mandino

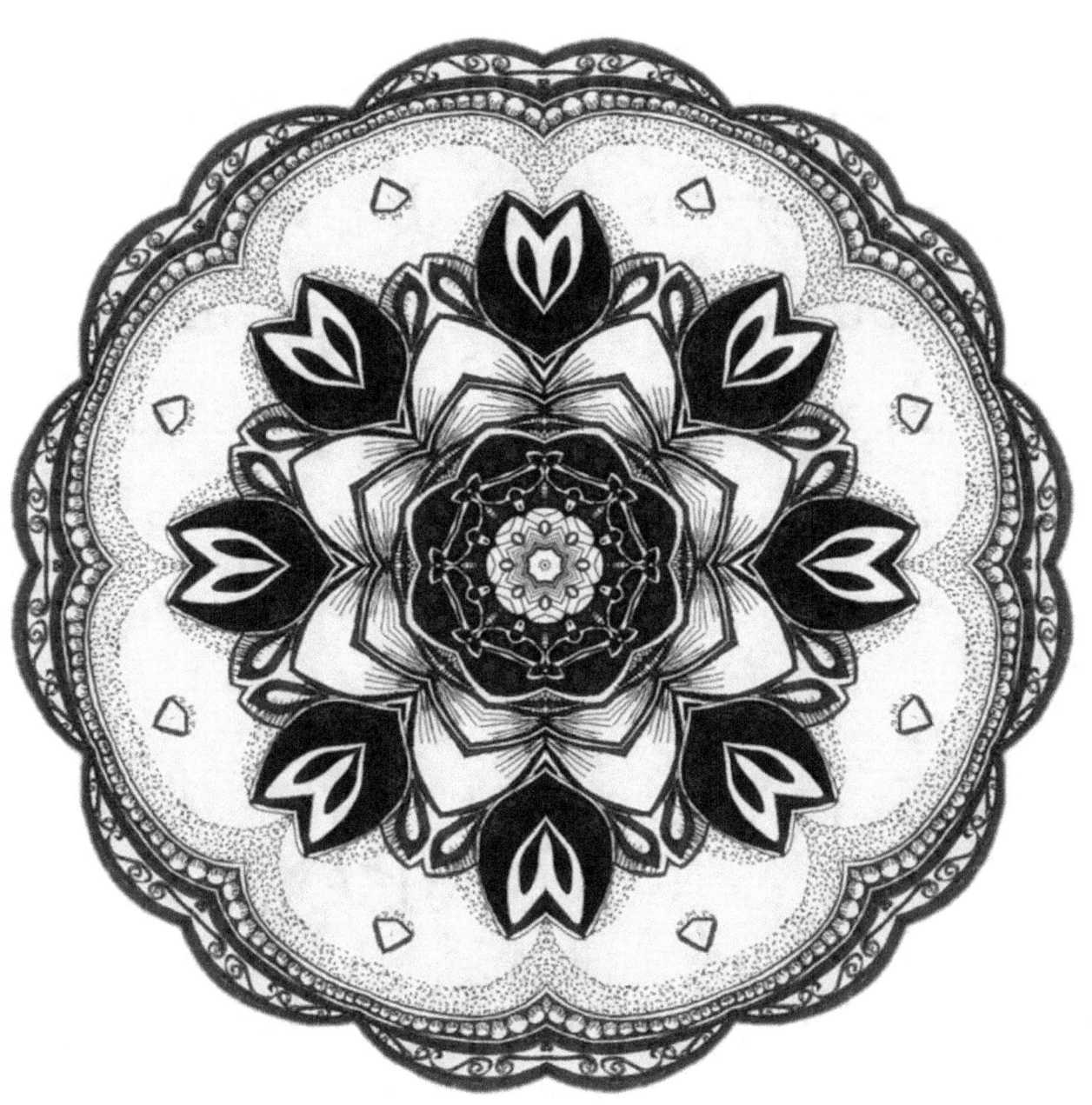

You know, all that really matters is that the people you love are happy and healthy. Everything else is just sprinkles on the sundae.

Paul Walker

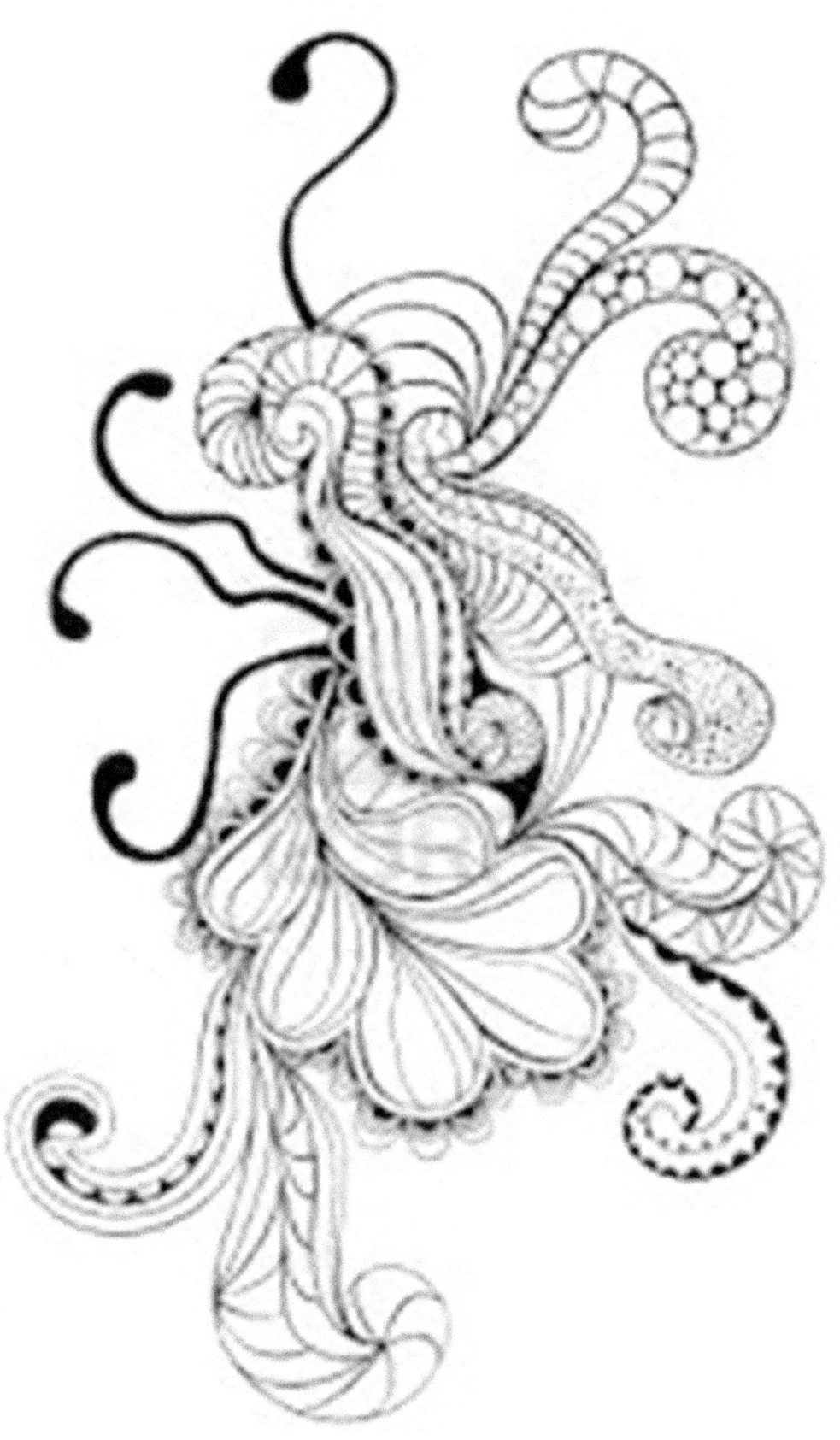

Natural forces within us are
the true healers of disease.

Hippocrates

Cheerfulness is the best promoter of health and is as friendly to the mind as to the body.

Joseph Addison

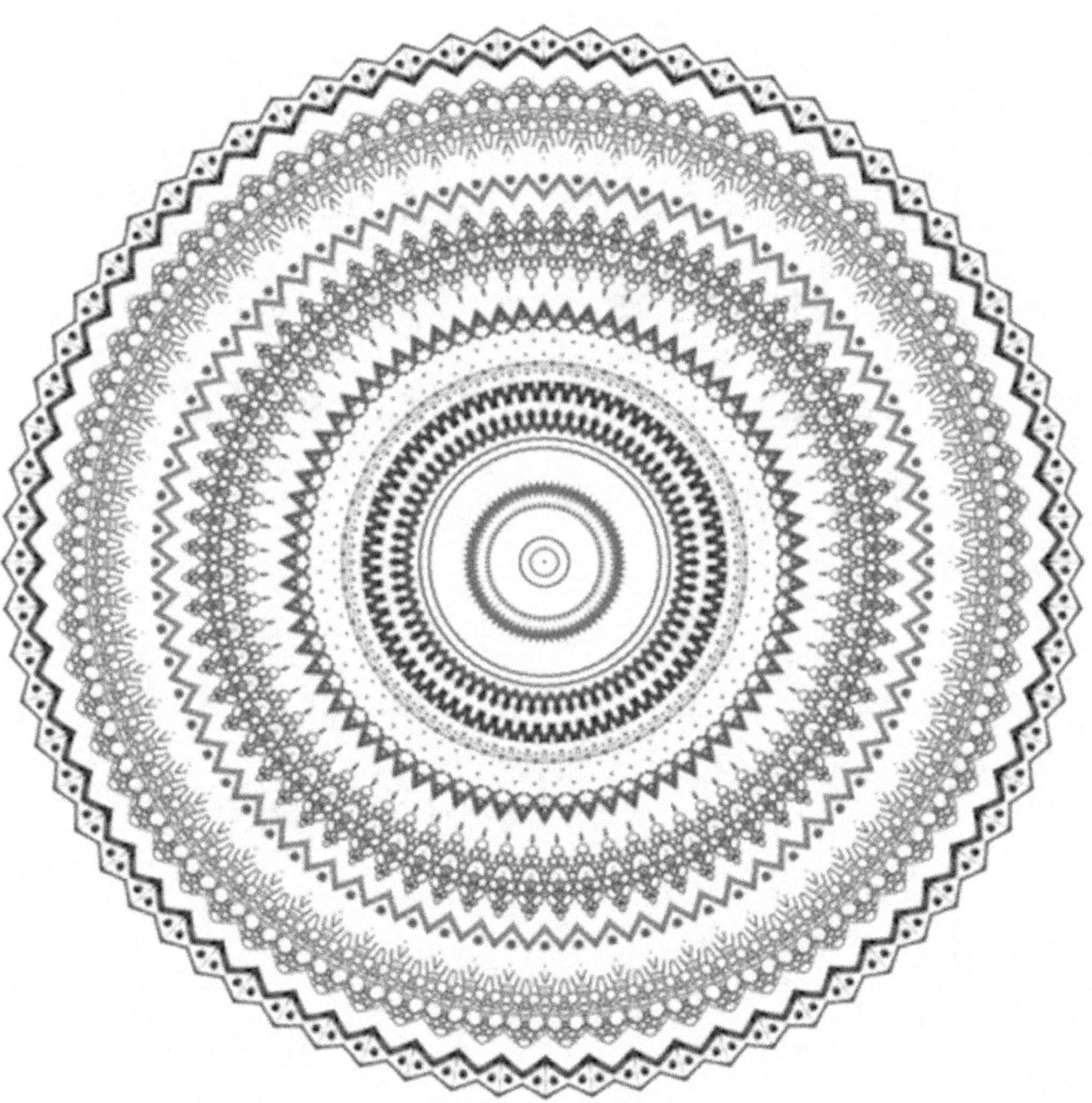

A healthy attitude is contagious but don't wait to catch it from others. Be a carrier.

Tom Stoppard

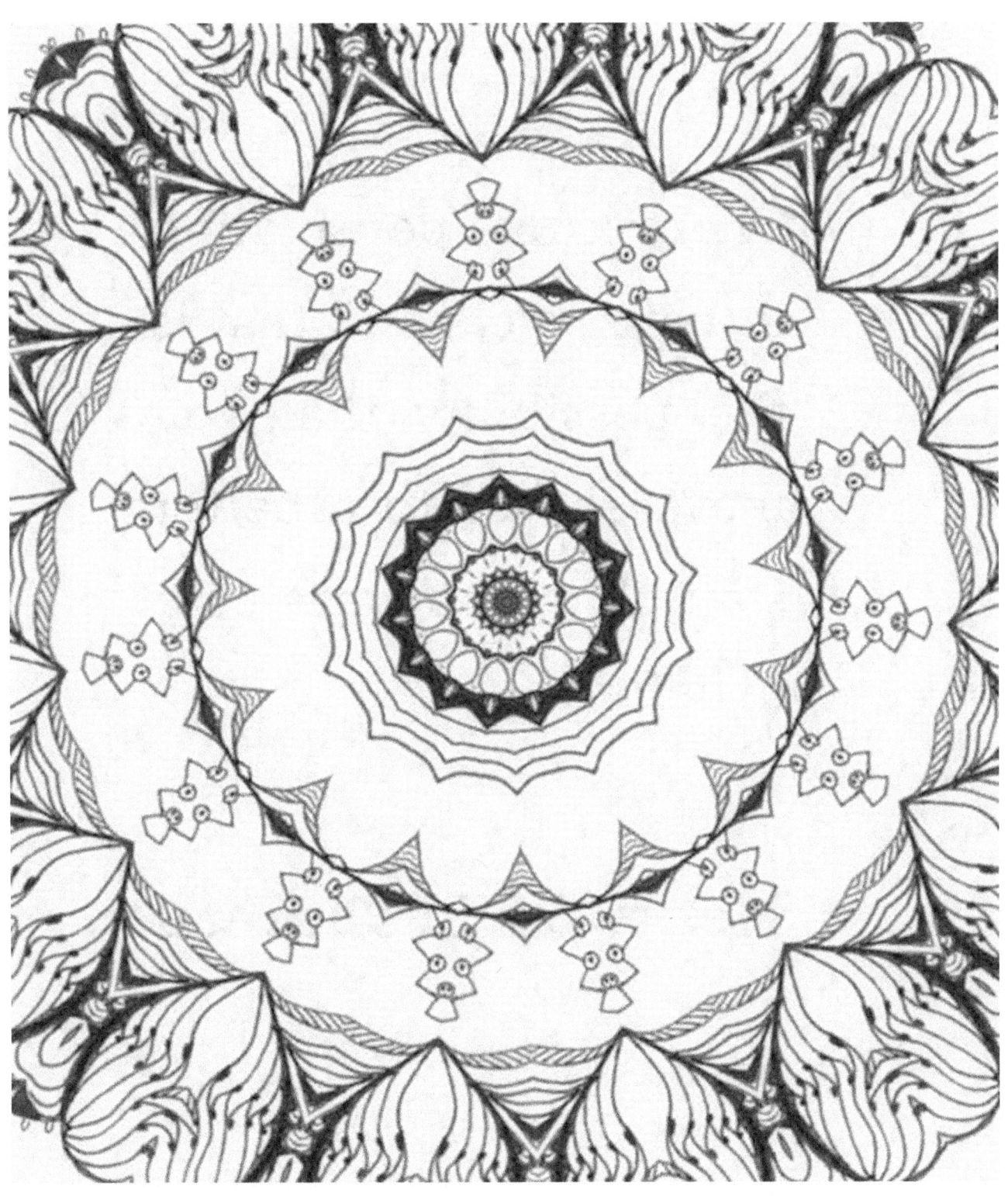

There is one consolation in being sick; and that is the possibility that you may recover to a better state than you were ever in before.

Henry David Thoreau

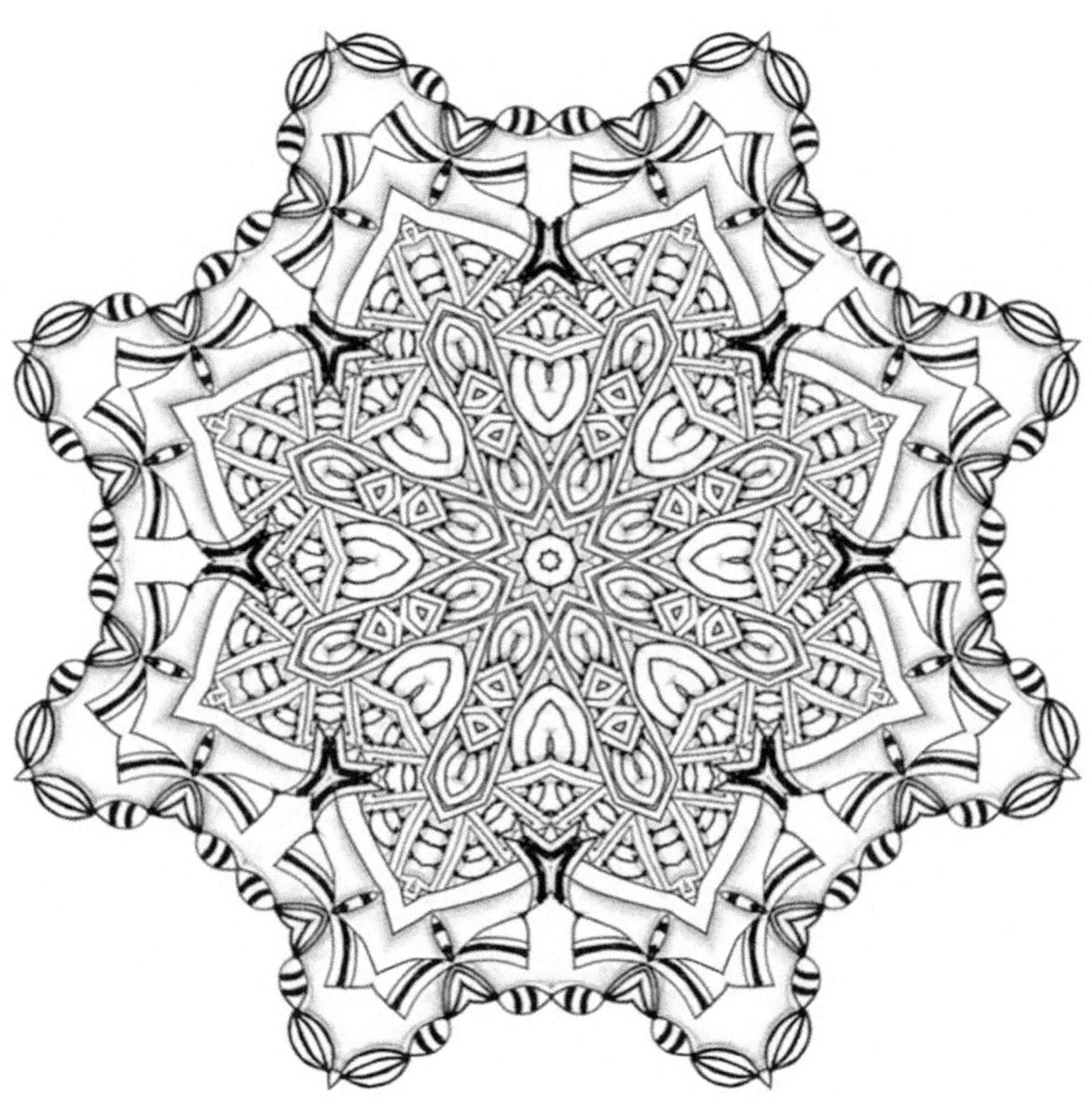

A healthy outside starts
from the inside.

Robert Urich

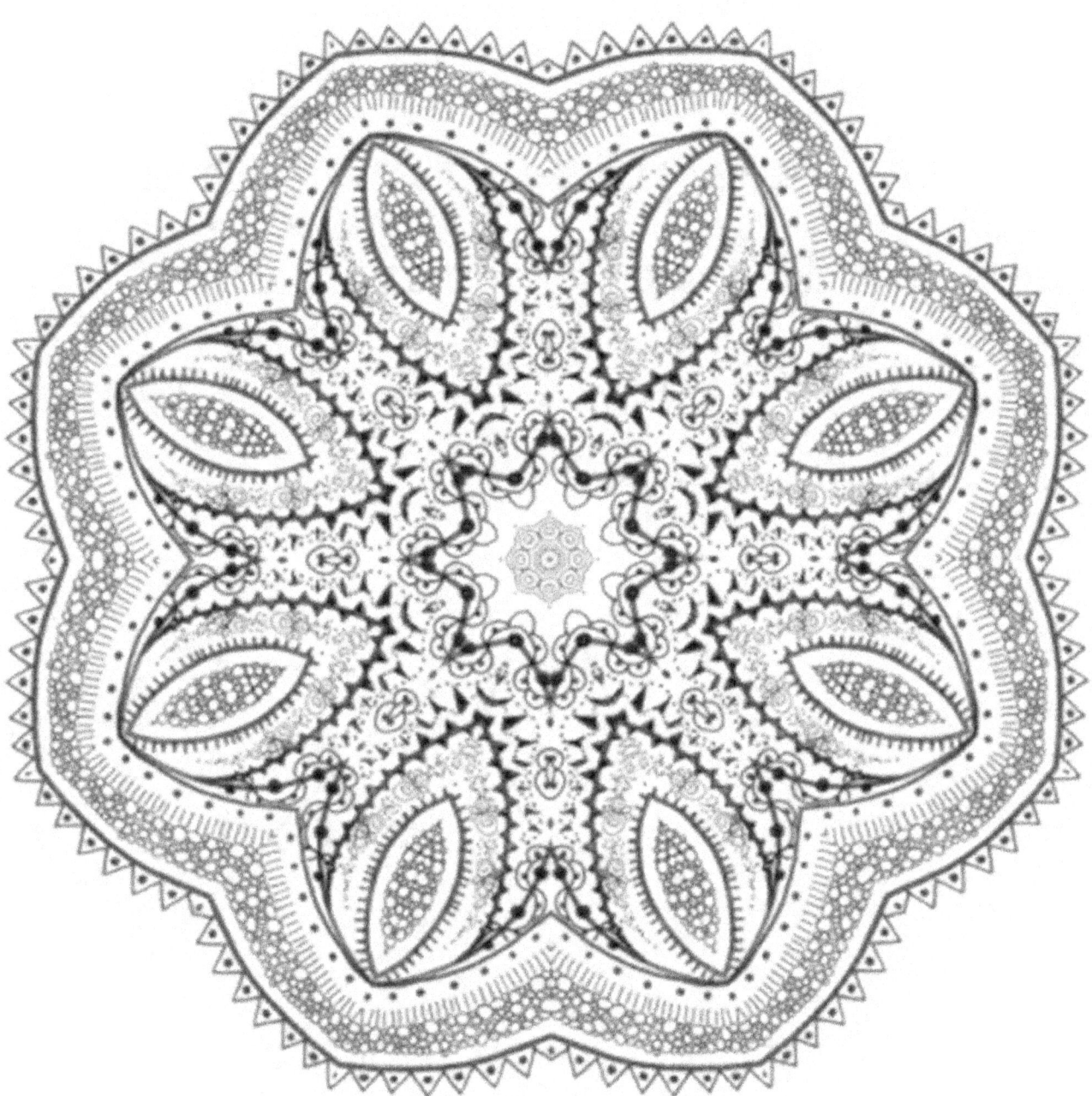

It takes more than just a good looking body. You've got to have the heart and soul to go with it.

Epictetus

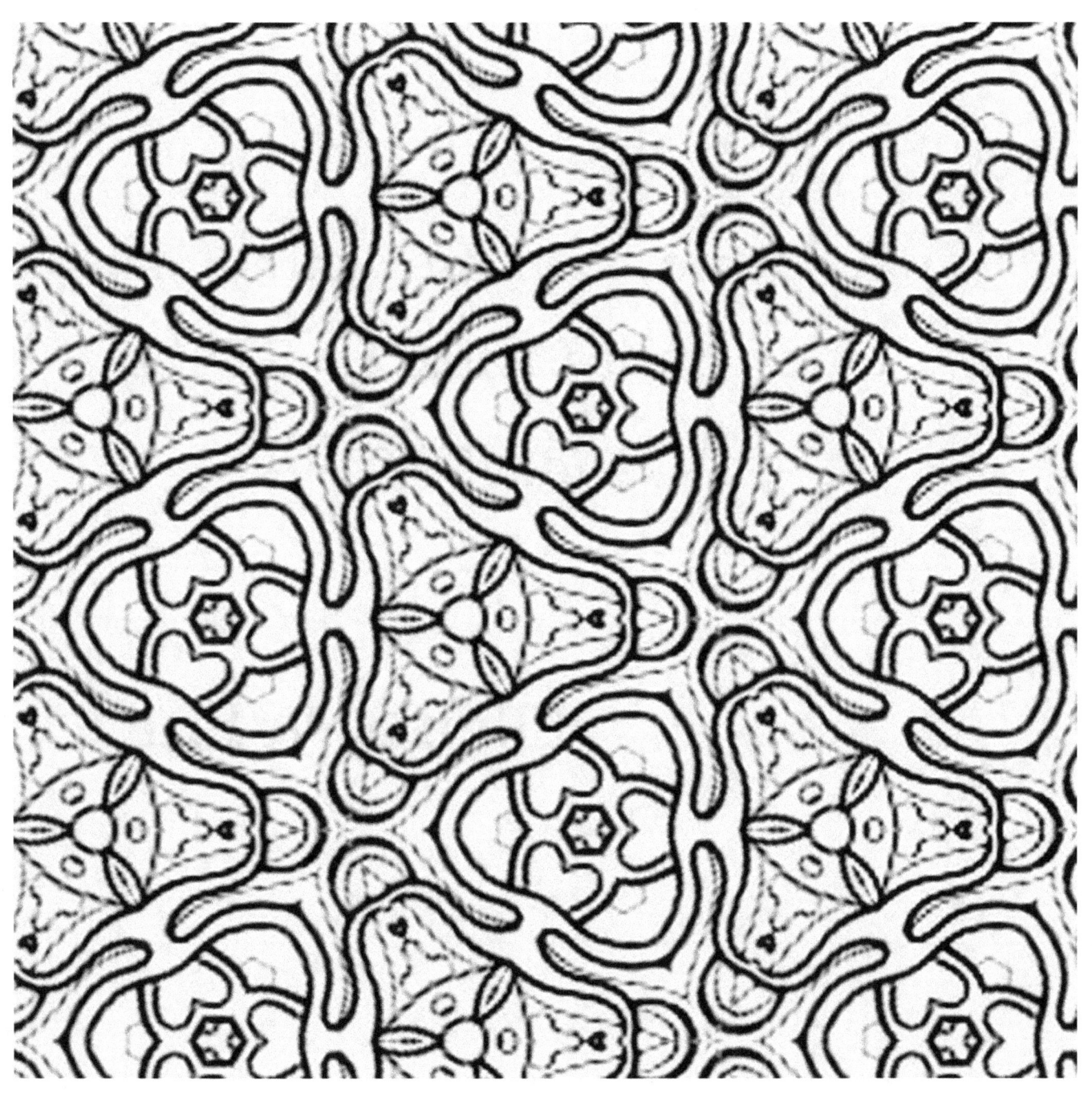

A person whose mind is quiet and satisfied in God is in the pathway to health.

Ellen G. White

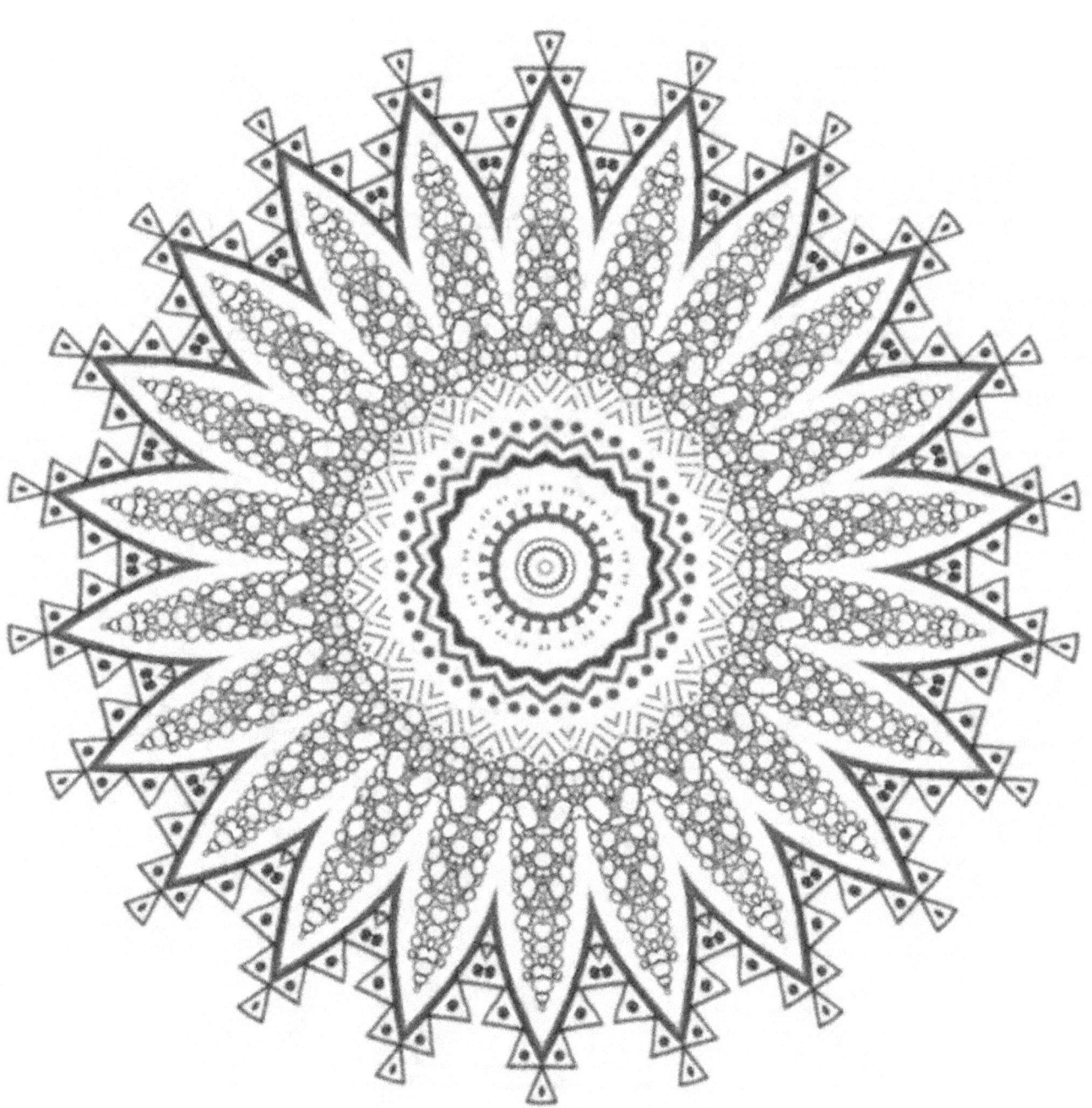

Healing is a matter of time, but it is sometimes also a matter of opportunity.

Hippocrates

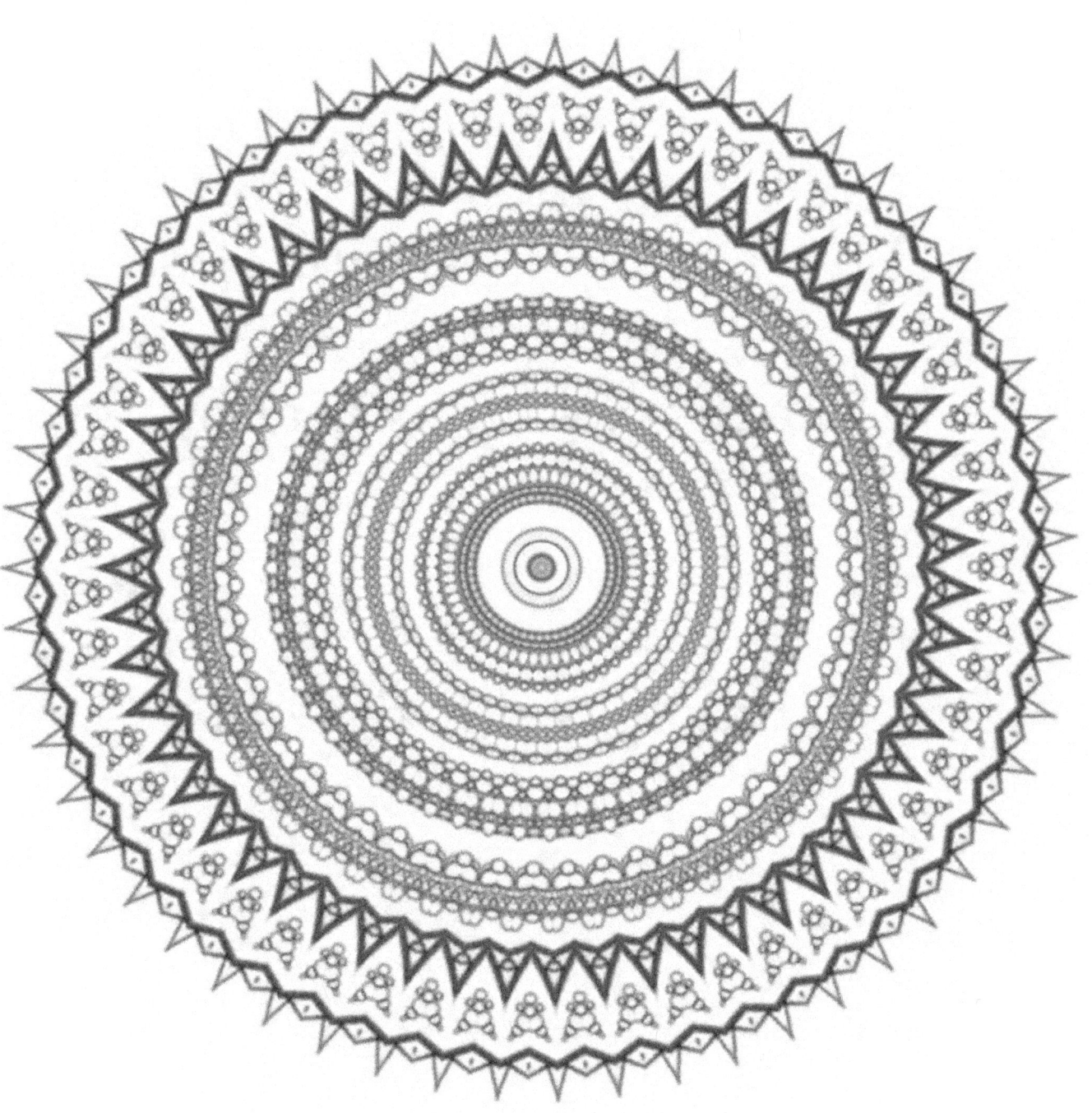

The first wealth is health.

Ralph Waldo Emerson

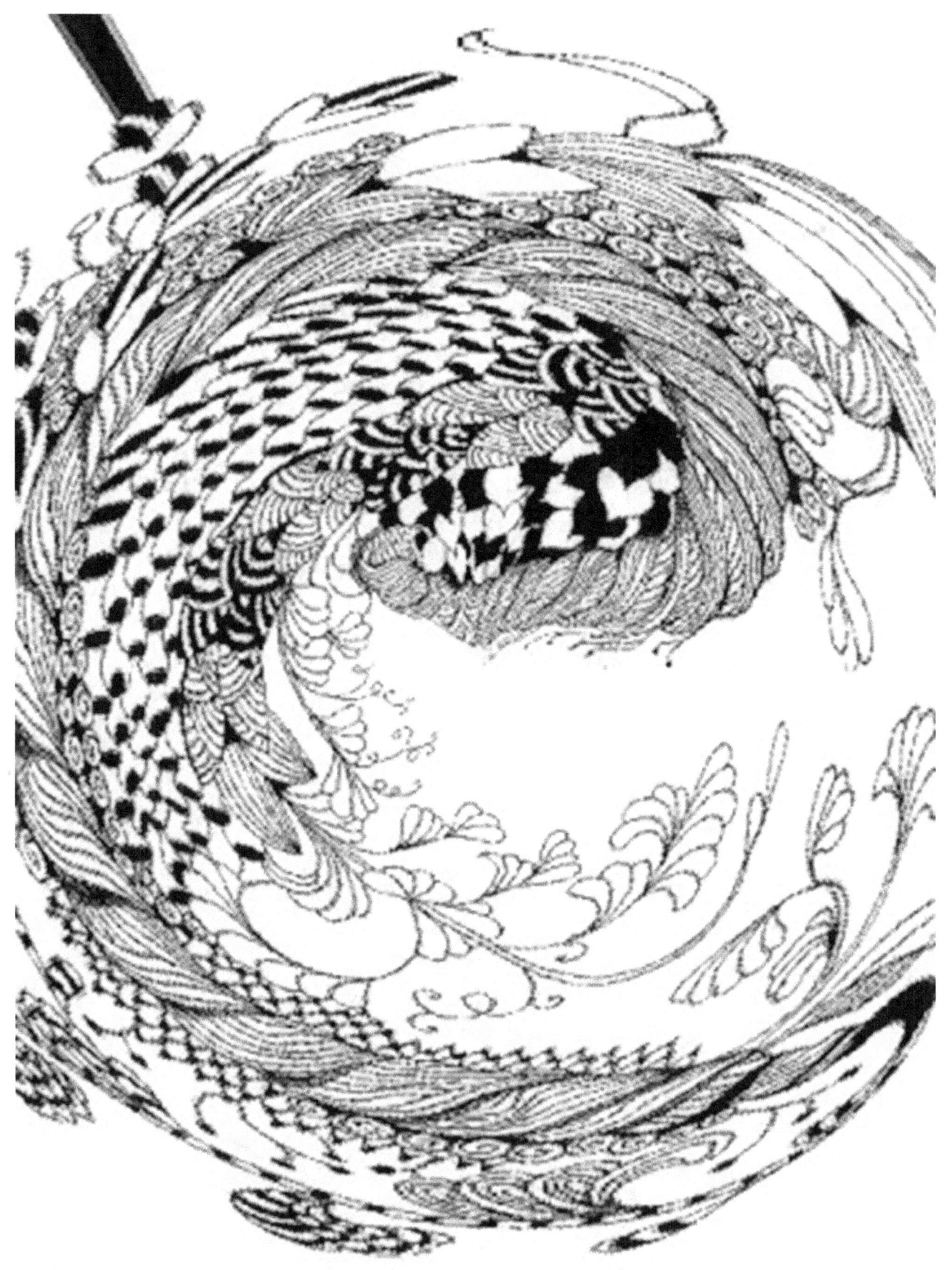

True silence is the rest of the mind, and is to the spirit what sleep is to the body, nourishment and refreshment.

William Penn

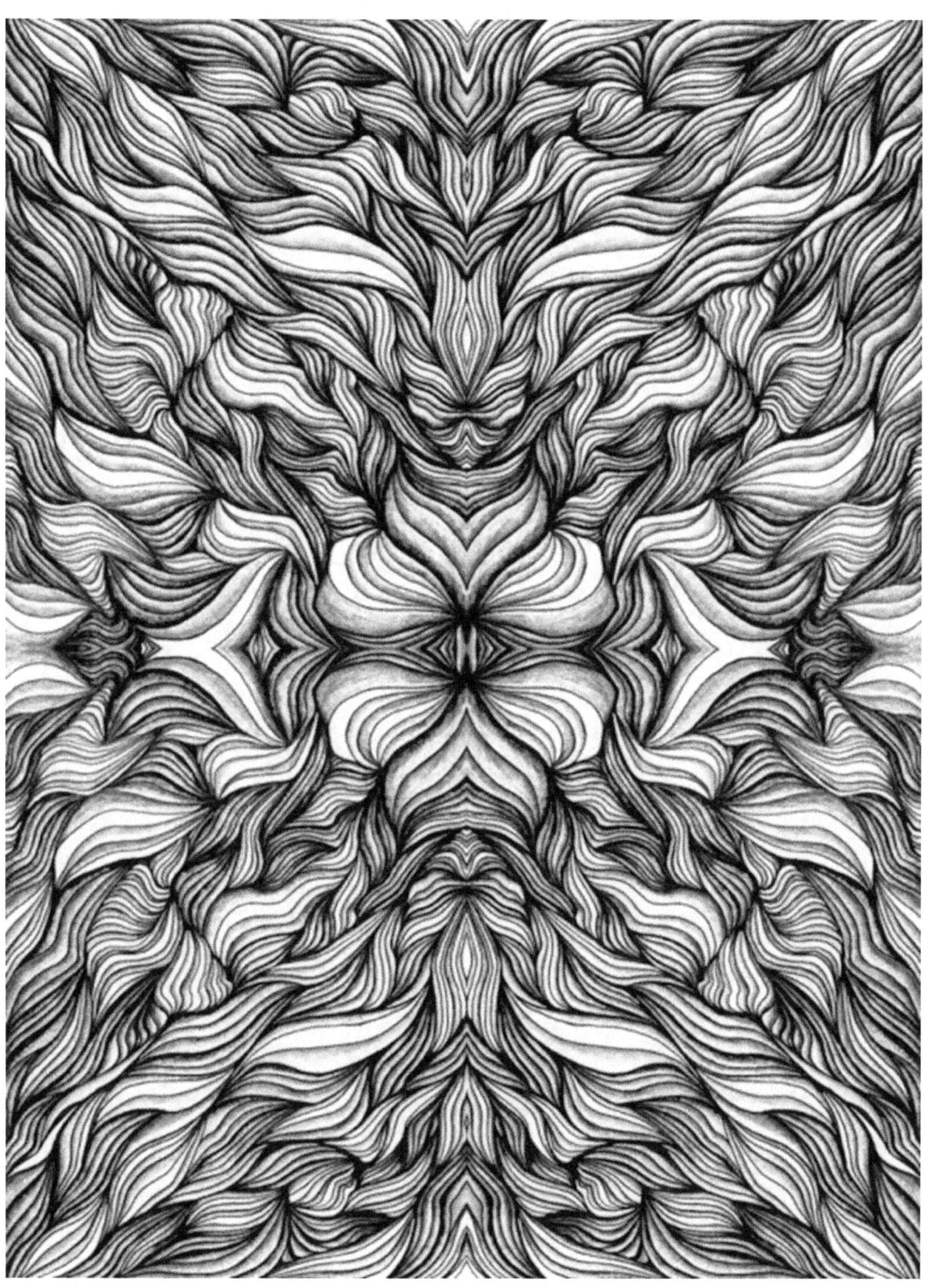

Hearty laughter is a good way to jog internally without having to go outdoors.

Norman Cousins

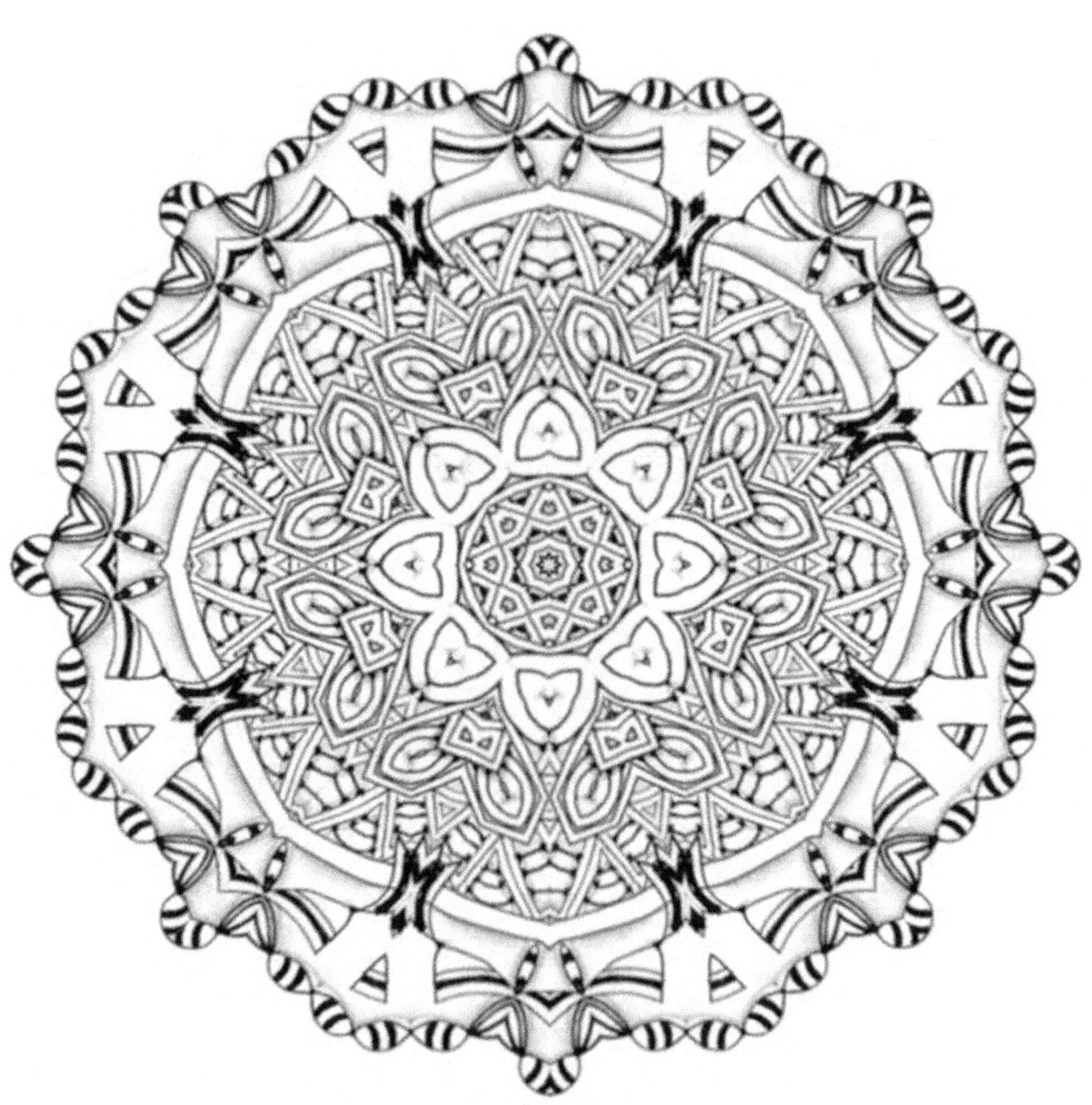

The way you think, the way you behave, the way you eat, can influence your life by 30 to 50 years.

Deepak Chopra

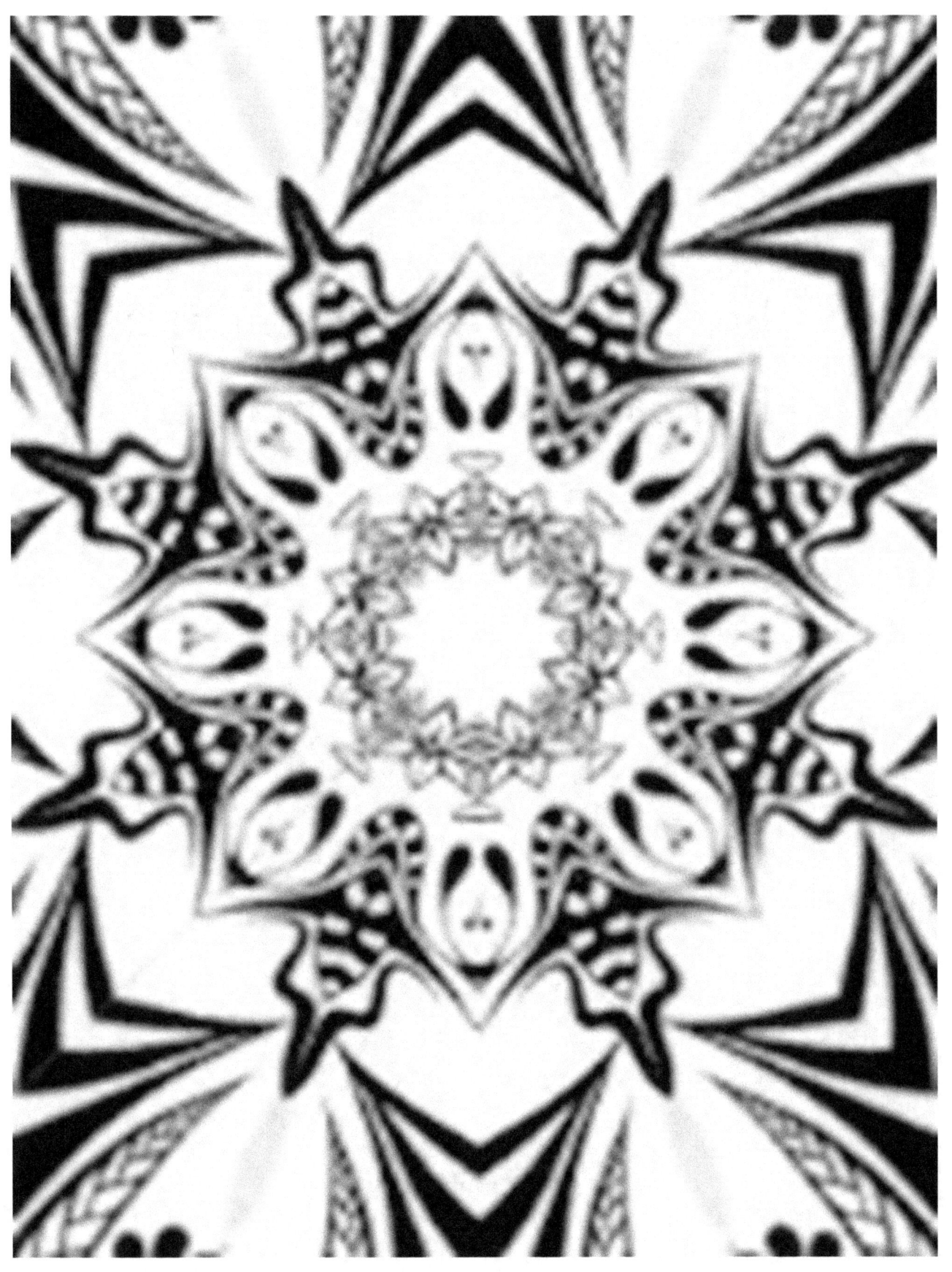

Be careful about reading health books. You may die of a misprint.

Mark Twain

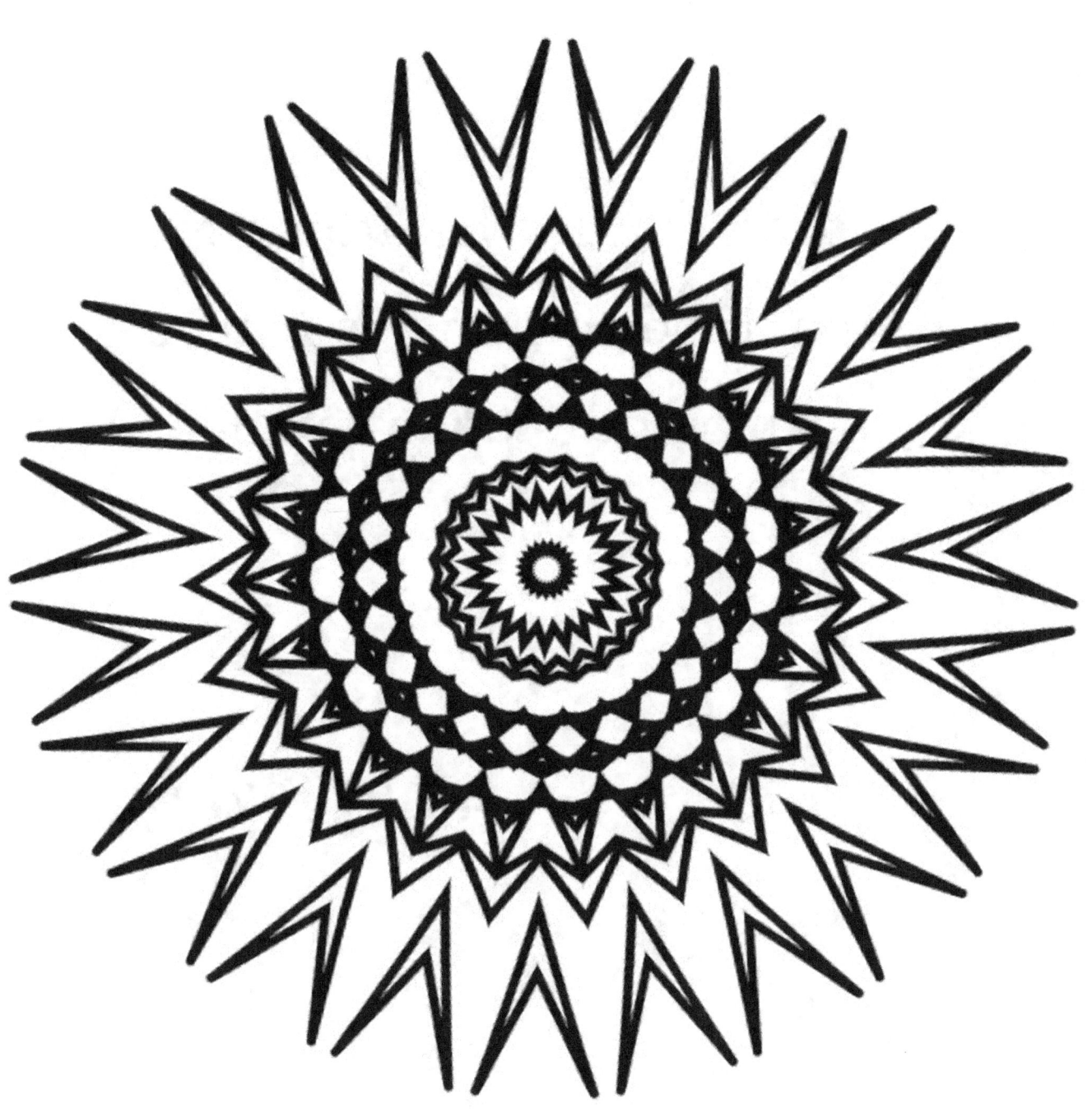

I find it a lot healthier for me to be someplace where I can go outside in my bare feet.

James Taylor

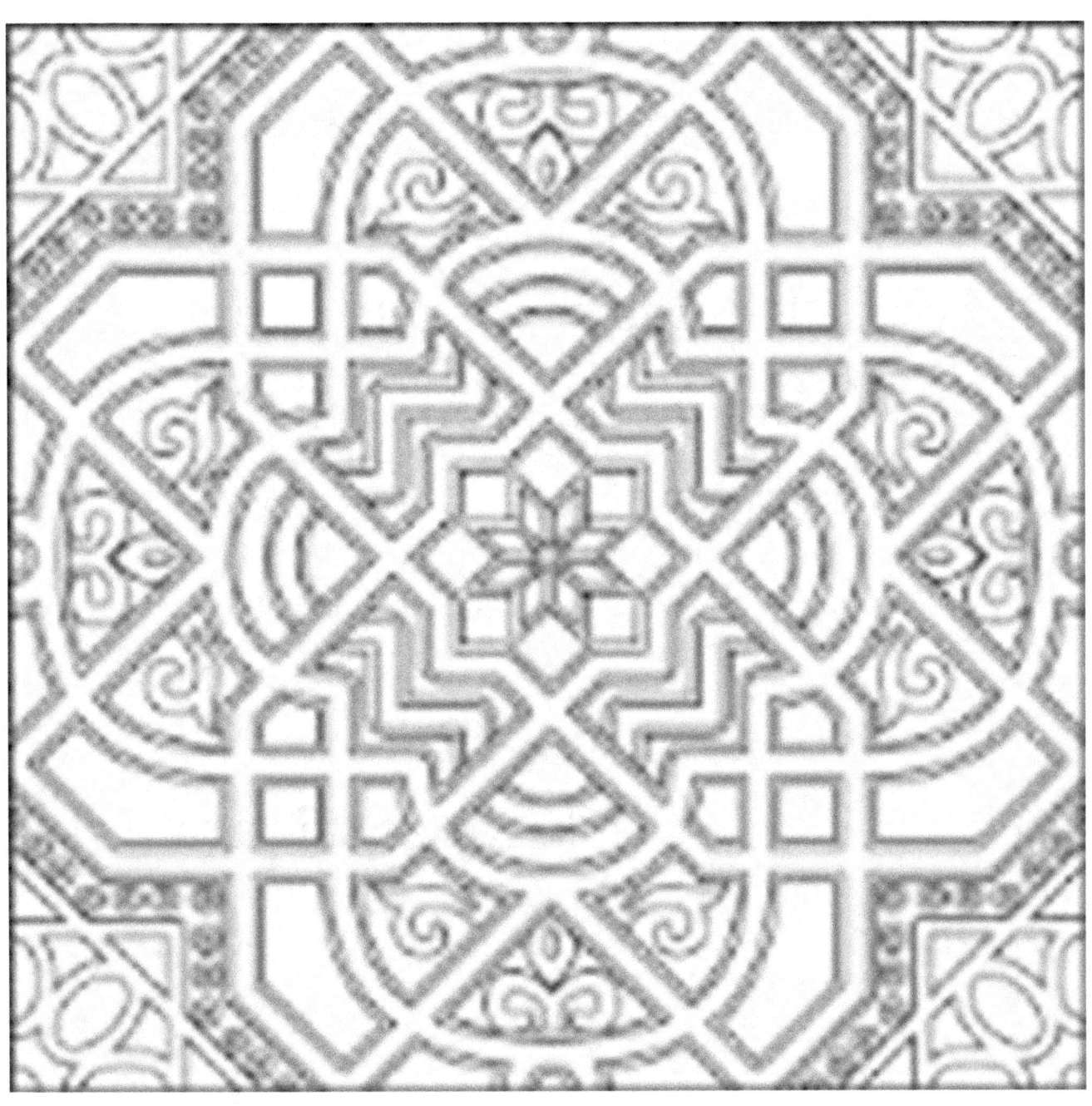

I pray God may preserve your health and life many years.

Junipero Serra

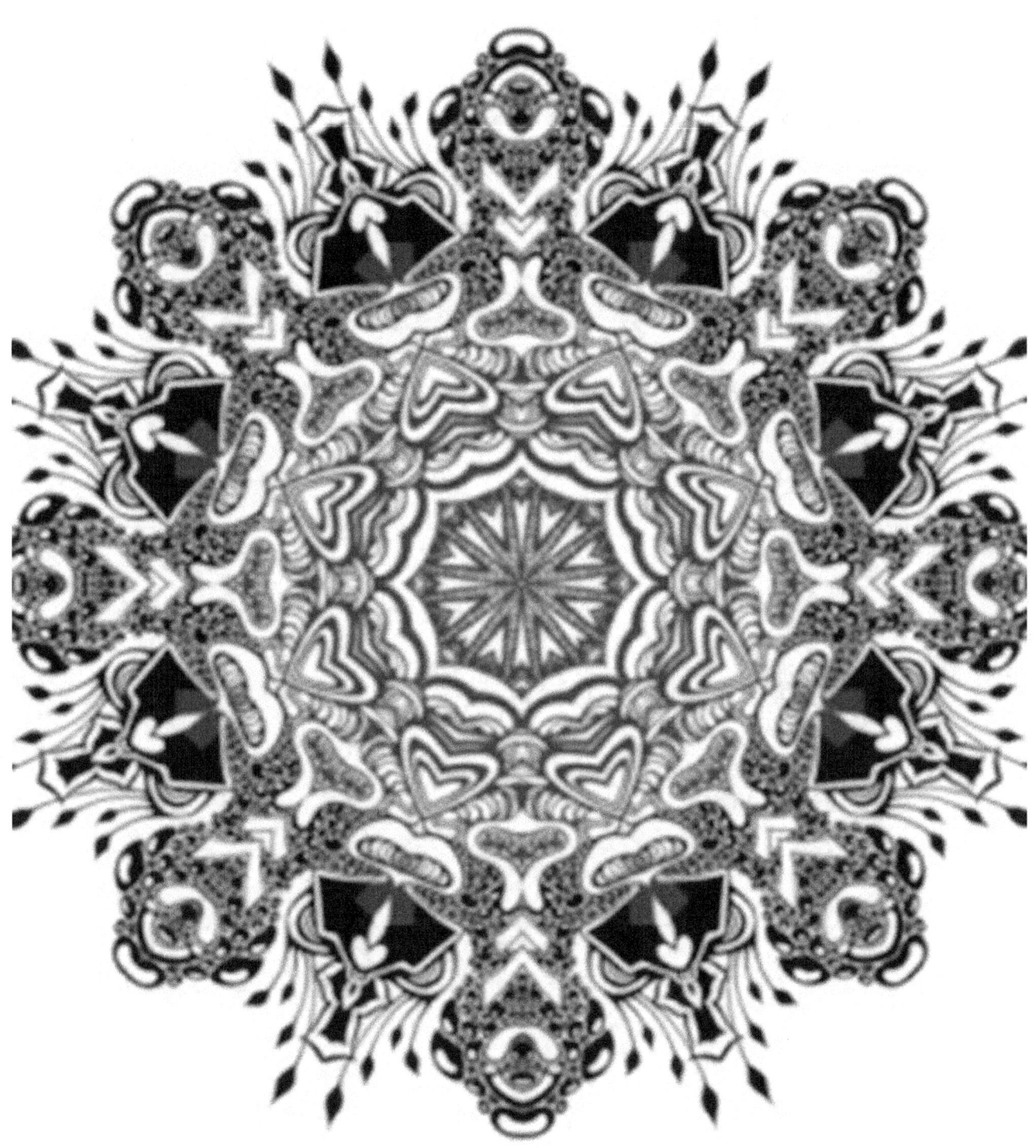

I believe that parents need to make nutrition education a priority in their home environment. It's crucial for good health and longevity to instil in your children sound eating habits from an early age.

Cat Cora

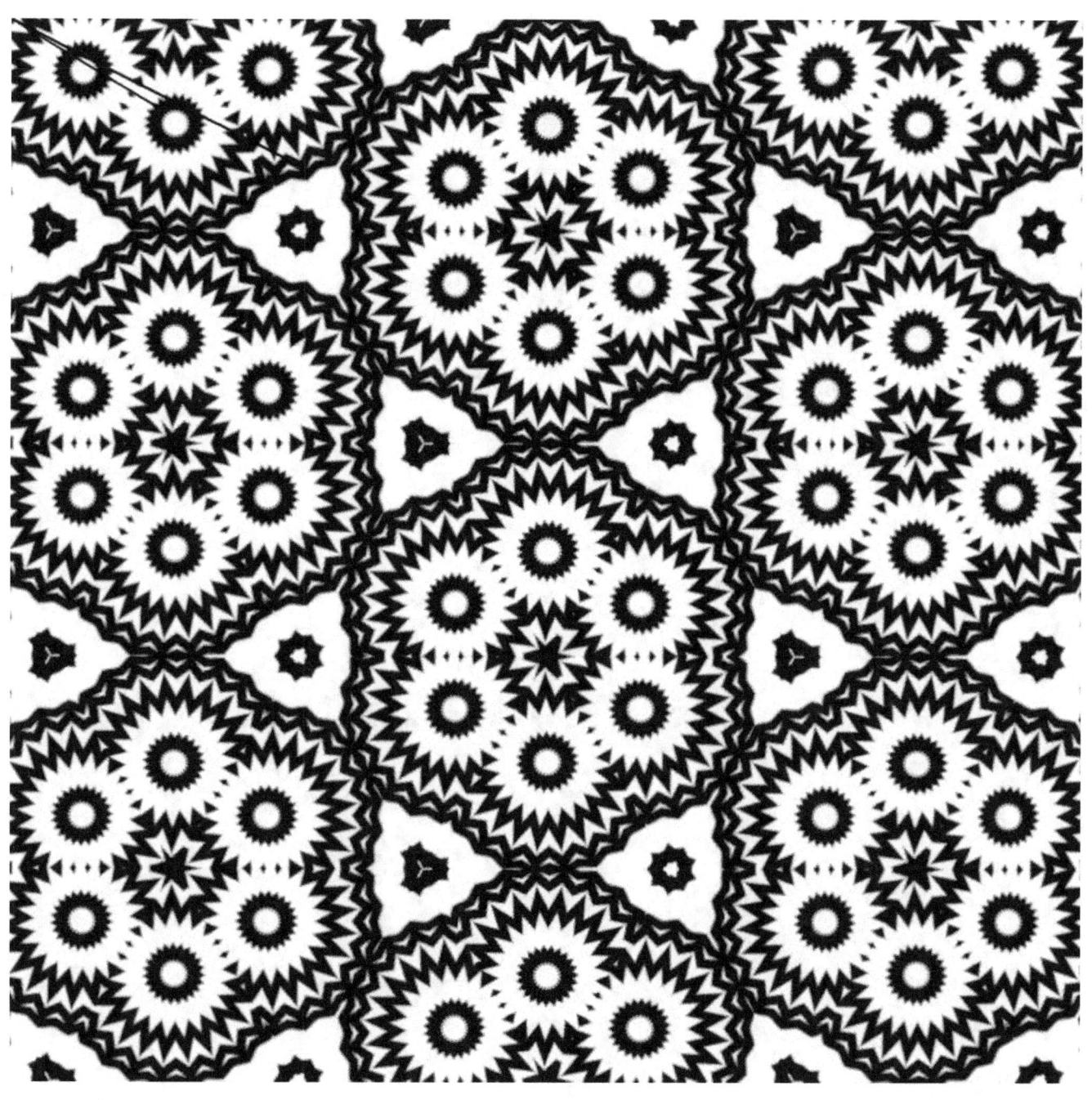

The world is mud-
luscious and puddle-
wonderful.

e. e. cummings

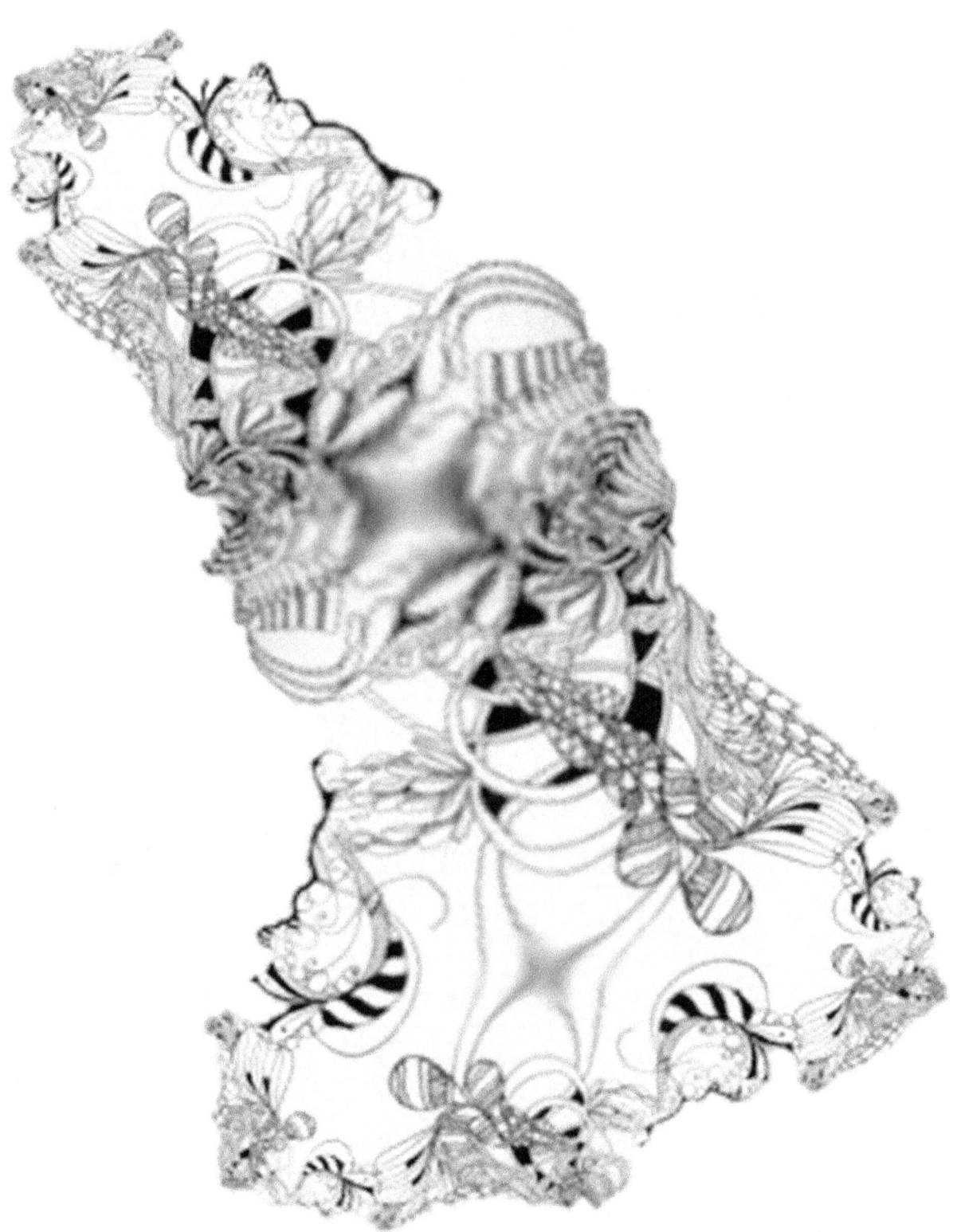

Yesterday is not ours to recover, but tomorrow is ours to lose.

Lyndon B Johnson

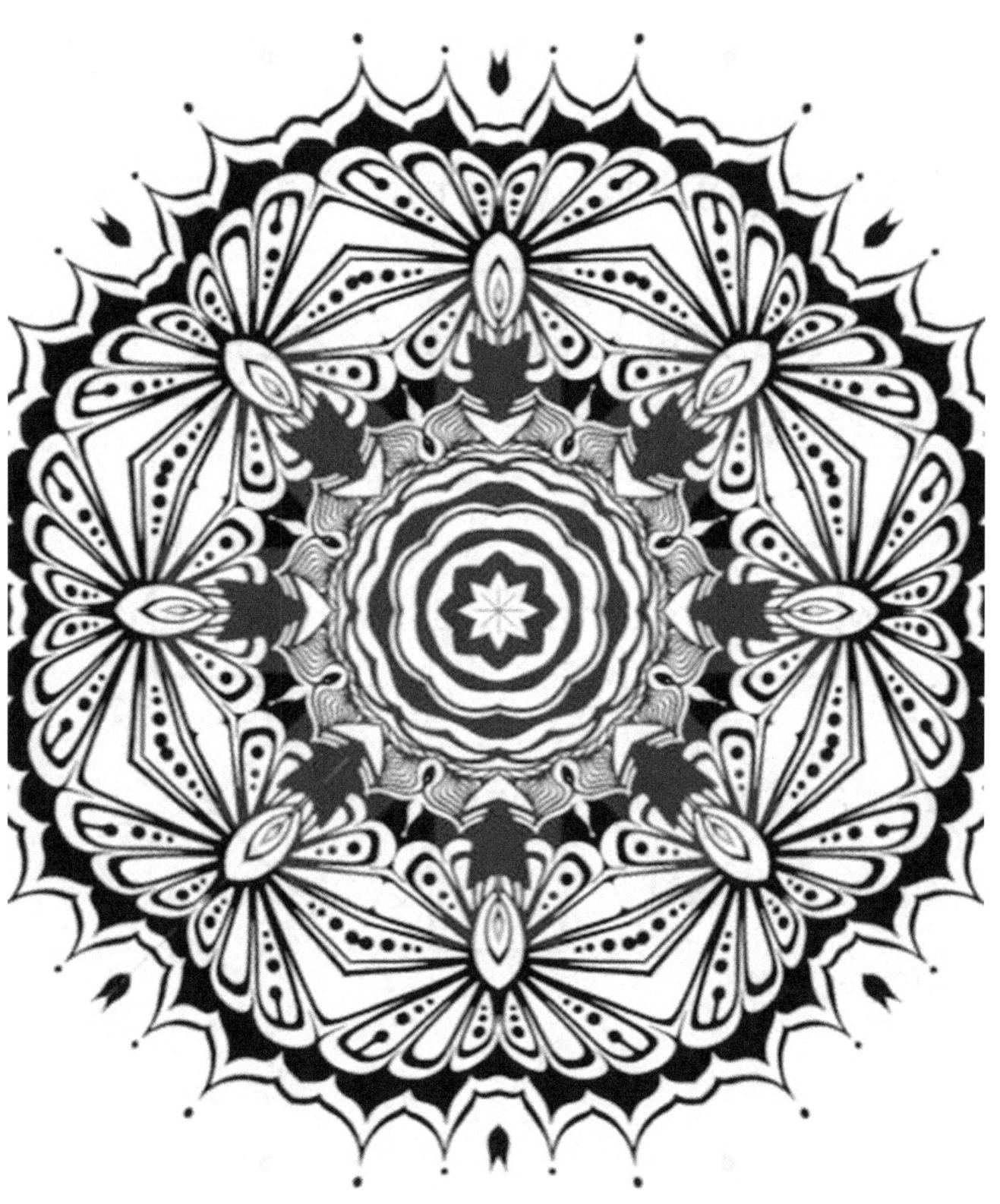

Thank you for your purchase.

If you enjoyed this book, then I'd like to ask you for a favour.

I will appreciate if you would leave a review for this book on Amazon. That will be greatly appreciated. Thank you in advance.

Also, if you had a very satisfying experience coloring this book, you may perhaps like to look at my other book (Alice in Wonderland Coloring Book) that can be accessed by going to the following link.

http://www.amazon.com.au/gp/product/B018JTBW7I

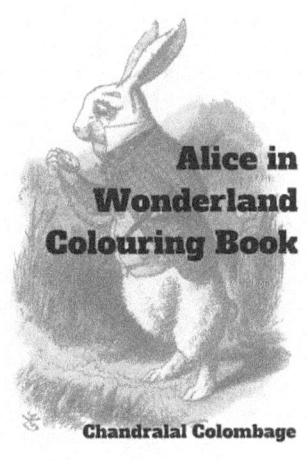

Alice in Wonderland Colouring Book

Chandralal Colombage